WELLNESS WARRIOR
MASTERCLASS SECRETS

WELLNESS WARRIOR MASTERCLASS SECRETS

9 Natural Cures & Holistic Healing Secrets
...NO ONE EVER TOLD YOU...

Noelle Powers

Legal Disclaimer:

Although Author and Publisher have made every effort to ensure that the information in this book was correct at press time, the Author and Publisher do hereby disclaim and do not assume any liability to any Party for any loss, damage or disruption caused by errors or omissions, resulting from negligence, accidents or any other cause.

This Book is not intended as a substitute for the medical advice of a Licensed Physician. The reader should always consult a Physician in matters relating to his/her heath, particularly with respect to any symptoms that may require diagnosis or medical attention.

The information in this Book is intended to supplement personal health care practices. The Author and Publisher advise readers to take full responsibility for their safety. Before practicing the methods revealed in this Book, be sure to have proper medical assessments performed on your current health condition. Do not take risks beyond your experience, ability or comfort level.

ISBN: 9798366261036
Copyright: © 2022 *Wellness Warrior*

Editor: *Noelle Powers*
Printed in the United States of America

This Book is dedicated to my Wonderful, Powerful Children.
They are my life's Triumph and Treasure.

To my Patient, Loving Sister who inspired me to write.

To God for blessing me with Wisdom to share.
For all Healings Past, Present and to Come, to Him goes the Glory.

I wish above all things that thou mayest Prosper and be in Health…"
3 John 2

Above all, the purpose of a Doctor is to awaken the Natural Healing Energies of the Body."
Hippocrates
420 B.C.

CONTENTS

Introduction

Congratulations on taking the first small yet powerful step towards making a critical change in your health and in your life.

Wellness Warrior is a Revelation. It reveals to you unique Alternative Healing Treatments born from the *rigors of Science* and the *Power and Wisdom of Nature*. It is a wellspring of *Uncommon Knowledge and Inspiration.* This book was written in the belief that it would radically improve peoples' health, not for a week or for a month, but for the rest of their lives. I believe that the first thing this book can do is *to cure fear, doubt and worry.* It can heal your feelings of helplessness. *If you are sick, you don't have to stay sick. If you are well, you don't have to worry about becoming sick. If your parents had Diabetes, Heart Disease or Alzheimer's, you don't have to fear that these things are therefore inevitable. You CAN absolutely take the wheel and turn down the path to Exceptional Health. All you need is the knowledge, the inspiration…and a MAP. This book gives you all three.*

For decades, I have experienced stunning results from the Natural Remedies you will discover here. Can I promise that every one of these methods will work for you exactly as they have worked for me? Well, I can promise you this: *Properly applying the knowledge in this book will make it exponentially more likely for you to Master your Health, for a lifetime.*

I am not a licensed Medical Doctor...which is precisely why you purchased this book. You are seeking safe, effective, alternative methods to regain and maintain your optimal health, which are outside the scope of traditional medicine. Giving all respect to the medical community, we must note that they are restricted to implementing a set, pre-approved list of protocols for whatever ailments you may have. You have purchased this book because, in part or in whole, these set protocols have not been successful for you.

Revealed in the 2003 Medical Report to Congress, prescription drug interactions and their negative side effects were the third leading cause of death in the U.S. So, choosing an effective Holistic Treatment whenever possible is usually a much safer alternative. If you know anyone who is stuck in the endless "prescription loop" yet they are not getting any better, *this is the path to a much better way.*

In truth, you are holding in your hand *the equivalent of 10 powerful booklets.*
Ten chapters that each reveal a separate, unique and detailed method of healing and achieving wellness. You can choose to use one protocol, or you can surely use them all to achieve your best possible vitality and well-being. You will discover health-changing protocols that are 4,000 years old, and some that are relatively new. The Testimonials will confirm that each one of these Natural Treatments has been successful at greatly alleviating, if not completely healing, a myriad of disorders for myself, my friends and my family.

The best results can only be achieved if the reader follows the very simple but exact instructions regarding each practice. For this reason, at the end of every chapter will be a section called *"Follow the Recipe"* which gives *3 easy to follow steps* showing exactly how to implement each Practice, optimizing the results of each Holistic Healing Method. You will discover what to *ADD* to your life, and just as importantly, what to *REMOVE* from it. After all, there's no use bailing water out of a sinking boat unless you first "*plug the holes in the boat*," correct?

For the past 30 years, I have voraciously researched and diligently compiled a wealth of knowledge on Natural Healing methods which cover an array of ailments. I drew this knowledge from decades of scientific evidence from foremost scientists, Nobel Prize Winners and world renowned experts who are much more educated in their field than I am. Just as importantly, I have spent my lifetime personally *applying this knowledge* and, for the most part, *succeeding* in the treatment of a wide range of disorders.

Now, I thought it was high time to share the wealth.

The beauty of this book is that you now have in your possession the *best of both worlds*: both the deluge of documented proof, as well as stunning testimonials from myself and others who have lived through each triumph. You will find these testimonials to be both fascinating and inspiring...*and best of all, they are TRUE.* I'm so excited to share each one with you.

Growing up in an Italian family, it was commonplace to hear the old Italian ladies declare, *"If you have your health, you have everything."* As a small child, I remember being increasingly annoyed each time I heard this constant chant. However, with adulthood came the revelation of the Wisdom that was in those words. Let me tell you...the day, the hour, the moment that your good health and vitality depart from you, those words ring loudly in your soul. How quickly do we then forage for healing and frantically pray for health's return. We immediately learn that life's joy and peace are firmly hinged upon having a vital, healthy body.

Good *Physical, Mental and Spiritual* health are the driving force of our lives. All must be in alignment to receive and enjoy the bounty of blessings Life has to offer. To balance these three factors is to *win the Trifecta* of a fulfilling and empowered Life. Although the Mind and Spirit have their own unique requirements for balance, I believe *once the Body is healed, the Mind and Spirit invariably partake in the Victory.*

To me, the journey of healing the Body seems to be the simplest of the three challenges, as the methods are quite black and white. There are health-damaging practices that must be removed from your daily habits, to be replaced with new choices which will breed good health. These will be clearly defined at the end of each chapter. Simply put, each "Action Recipe" is like baking a cake. *For best results, we must follow the simple "Recipe for Healing," without omissions or substitutions.*

To adapt to each person's learning style, I have structured every chapter to contain subsections. Readers like me who wish to know the history and scientific proof of each treatment can enjoy the science and history section of each chapter. Conversely, those readers that *are not interested* in the scientific data *can skip that section* and move forward to other categories within each chapter. This should delight those of you that may not care *how each treatment works;* you're just happy *that it works.* Now, for *the "just give me the short version"* readers, I have interpolated many *Bullet Points* which succinctly define the gist of each chapter. Lastly, you will enjoy extraordinary stories and testimonials which exemplify the astonishing results that each one of these Natural Healing habits has achieved.

Whether we call these practices Alternative Medicine, Holistic Healing or Natural Cures, Naturopathic Remedies, they are all under the same umbrella of lifetime Optimal Health.

As you practice each unique method, you are not only teaching yourself how to achieve wellness, but you are *mastering knowledge* that will enable you to maintain optimal health for the rest of your life. In turn, you can help those you love to do the same. So let's dip into this *Well of Wisdom* together. As a reward for yourself, and as
a Legacy of Wellness for your children.

At this very moment,
       Your Health is in your Hands.

              So, strap yourself in
                   ...and let the Journey begin...

Chapter One

"THE TREE OF LIFE"
Raw, Unrefined Coconut Oil

What if I told you...
That there is an all-natural food which:

> Resuscitates dying brain cells,
> Lowers cholesterol, kills viruses, bacteria, fungus and parasites in your body,
> Supports your thyroid and increases your metabolism,
> Improves brain, eye and cardiovascular health,
> Strengthens your immune system,
> Prevents Alzheimer's and reverses symptoms
> Prevents Diabetes and reverses symptoms
> Promotes weight loss,
> ...and that it tastes a lot like butter...?

Are you in...?

That food is raw, unrefined Coconut Oil.
I believe it is the single most valuable health food treasure you will ever find.

Says Who...?
Dr. George Blackburn, Harvard Medical School Researcher, Mary G. Enig, Ph.D. Biochemist; Dr. Trowbridge, President of the American College for the Advancement of Medicine; Dr. Julian Whitaker from the

world famous Whitaker Wellness Center; Dr. Ray Peat, Ph.D. Endocrinologist; Dr. Jon Kabara, Professor of Chemistry and Pharmacology at Michigan State University; Dr. Bruce Fife, C.N., N.D. and literally hundreds more scientists and researchers whose list of names would give you a headache to read. After exhaustive studies, these esteemed professionals who are experts in their field comprise the All-Star Cast who agree that all of the above...*is true.*

Dr. Bruce Fife is a certified Nutritionist and Doctor of Naturopathic Medicine. He serves as the Publisher of Piccadily Books/Health Wise Publications and has written 18 books on achieving good health.

A multitude of health-changing facts about Coconut Oil are documented in Dr. Fife's Book *The Coconut Oil Miracle* and in Dr. Mary Newport's Book *Alzheimer's Disease, What if There Was a Cure?* You will also learn crucial discoveries proven and documented by Dr. Weston A. Price, renowned for his 25-year extensive research on how dietary fat affects the health of native cultures around the world. His research has been confirmed many times over through studies done by a myriad of Scientists and Health Institutions over many decades of time. Their startling revelations and science-backed confirmations are included in the following pages. I am also adding to this my own personal Coconut Oil success stories and amazing testimonials.

How Does Coconut Oil Kill Microbes (germs)...?

An outer coating of fat encapsulates most bacteria and viruses. Picture a water balloon. This outer fatty cell wall is usually soft and fluid, composed of loosely attached fatty acids. This allows these damaging organisms to squeeze through the tiniest of openings. Coconut Oil is rich in *Medium Chain Fatty Acids* (MCFA's) which are the "Good Fats" that heal. These MCFA's in Coconut Oil are very small which makes it easy for them to penetrate the microbe's cell wall. They then cause that cell wall to weaken to such a degree that *it just disintegrates*. The microbe's outer membrane literally just splits open, spilling its insides and killing the organism. The cellular debris that spills out is then cleaned up by our white blood cells. This is how the MCFA's in Coconut Oil easily kill invading microorganisms in our body while causing no harm to surrounding healthy cells. The Science behind this power is both simple and amazing.

MCFA's are such an effective line of defense against microbes, that even our own bodies manufacture a small amount of it found in the oil secreted by our sebaceous (oil) glands on our skin. This very thin layer of oil helps protect us from the multitude of germs we come in contact with each day.

Supporting Science:
Health-Giving Effects of Raw Coconut Oil...
Dr. Conrado Dayrit, Professor Emeritus of Pharmacology University of Philippines and past President of National Academy of Sciences and Technology, held in-depth clinical studies which led to the breakthrough discovery that the Medium Chain Fatty Acids/MCFA's in Coconut Oil, specifically *Lauric and Capric Acid*, were nature's most potent antimicrobial, even effective in killing HIV in lab cultures.

Dr. Jon Kabara, Ph.D. Professor Emeritus Department of Chemistry and Pharmacology Michigan State University, was one of the first to discover the *Antimicrobial properties of MCFA's,* which are the essence of Coconut Oil. *He has been awarded 16 patents and has written eight books and more than 200 scientific publications.* Many of his peers judge him to be one of the foremost authorities on dietary fats.

Nature's Most Powerful Antimicrobial...

Coconut Oil is composed of several health-giving MCFA's. One of them, *Lauric Acid, was discovered* to *be antifungal, as well as antibacterial, antiviral and anti-parasitic.* This amazing discovery was first made by Dr. Jon Kabara in 1966. Dr. Kabara further confirmed that *48% of the MCFA's in Coconut Oil is Lauric Acid. This is the <u>highest amount of this potent antimicrobial found in any food</u>.* You might say it would be one stop shopping to include raw Coconut Oil in your daily diet, to help eliminate and prevent colonies of parasites, bacteria and viruses from slowly and silently growing inside your body. *Comprising nearly 50% of its fat content,* Coconut Oil is by far Nature's richest source of *Lauric Acid.* In Africa and Malaysia, Palm Kernel Oil (NOT to be confused with Palm Oil) comes in second. Mother's Milk has 6% *Lauric Acid,* while whole milk and butter have only 3%. These are the only food sources containing any significant amount of *Lauric Acid, Nature's most powerful antimicrobial.*

- *Lauric Acid, was discovered* to *be antifungal, as well as antibacterial, antiviral and anti-parasitic. Raw Coconut Oil is the highest food source of Lauric Acid.*

- *Please note that processed vegetable oils are completely deficient in Lauric Acid and other important MCFA's.*

- *Simply replacing all other oils in your kitchen with Coconut Oil is a simple choice that will have a profound impact on the improvement of your health.*

MICROORGANISMS KILLED BY MCFA'S IN COCONUT OIL :

Lipid coated viruses

Lipid coated bacteria

Lipid coated viruses	Lipid coated bacteria
Visna virus	Listeria monocytogenes
Cytomegalovirus	Helicobacter pylori
HIV	Haemophilus influenzae
Epstein-barr virus	Staphylococcus aureus
Influenza virus	Streptococcus agalactiae
Leukemia virus	GroupsA,B,F,&G streptococci
Pneumonia virus	Gram-positive organisms
Hepatitis C virus	Gram-negative organisms
Measles virus	(if treated with chelator)
Herpes simplex virus	Meningitis (neisseria)
Sarcoma virus	Chlamydia pneumonia
Syncytial virus	Propionibacterium acnes (acne)
Human lymphotropic virus (type I)	Chlamydia trachomatis
Vesicular stomatitis virus (VSV)	Pseudomonas Aeruginosa
	Acinetobacter baumannii

The native cultures of South and Central America relied upon Coconut Oil to maintain their health in an environment infested with malaria, yellow fever and other tropical diseases. In the Somalian and Ethiopian regions of Africa, the natives used Coconut Oil to stop seizures in their babies. Natives of South Pacific Islands, Panama and Jamaica used Coconut Oil as both a heart tonic and a cure. Even China has 2,000 year old Coconut Oil medical recipes which are recorded as "*cures for 69 diseases.*"

I once met a woman who was the healer in her village in West Africa. She advised she would put drops of raw Coconut Oil into the eyes and mouth of babies, as well as via enema, to stop seizures and heal them of a plethora of disorders. Since there are no known negative side effects for this kind of treatment, this was a safe and successful healing protocol which was passed down for generations in her family and in her village.

What Say the Researchers…?

Dr. Weston A. Price, D.D.S. is well known for having traveled the world for decades performing exhaustive research on the health and diet of native cultures. He has written a vast number of medical reports and books revealing in great detail that wherever the Coconut Palm grew, Coconut Oil was relied upon for that culture's health and healing. Among his many discoveries was the fact that in cultures, like South Pacific Islands and Polynesia the following was true:

- *Although their diet consisted of 60% saturated (good) fat from raw Coconut Oil, Native Cultures were virtually FREE from heart disease and other degenerative diseases. Dr. Price discovered these natives had clear arteries, well-formed bones, healthy hearts and strong healthy teeth with virtually no cavities.*

- *He further confirmed that, contrary to medical propaganda, all cultures which ate a diet high in this "good saturated fat" had NO high cholesterol, nor obesity nor hardening of the arteries.*

Early explorers described these cultures as being *exceedingly strong, vigorously built and beautiful in body.* Pacific Islanders traditionally ate copious amounts of coconuts and Coconut Oil every day. Yet they enjoyed lives virtually free from heart disease and other degenerative diseases which commonly plague the Western populations. It is because of its age-old litany of preventative and restorative benefits, that many cultures referred to the Coconut Palm as *"The Tree of Life."*

Pukapuka and Tokelau Island Study:

One of many extensive studies done on the effect of a *high good fat diet* was the Pukapuka and Tokelau Island study. This long-term study was done in the 1960s and included the entire population of both islands, approximately 2,500 people. Pukapuka and Tokelau are among the more isolated Polynesian islands. Having been isolated from Western dietary influence, they were the perfect case study.

Scientist Ian Prior led the study of the two island populations. The standard diet on both islands was a high-fat diet derived from coconuts and raw Coconut Oil. His records reflect that the average dietary fat intake was as high as *50% of their total daily calories from raw Coconut Oil,* yet this extensive study confirmed Dr. Price's findings: both populations *exhibited low cholesterol.* Also, they *were virtually free* from all heart disease, kidney disease, hypothyroidism, diabetes, colitis, hemorrhoids, ulcers, diverticulitis, and appendicitis. He recorded his final conclusions, as follows: *"Vascular disease is uncommon in both populations and there is no evidence of this high saturated fat intake having any harmful effect on these populations."*

- *In this study of 2,500 people whose daily diet consisted of 50% good saturated fat from Coconut Oil, it was confirmed that they had low cholesterol and were virtually free of heart disease, hypothyroidism, high blood pressure, arteriosclerosis and diabetes and kidney disease.*

The Kitava Study:

In the 1990s, another series of studies were done, known as the Kitava Study. The research was done on the health and diet of the South Pacific people on the Island of Kitava near Papua New Guinea. Staffan Lindeberg, M.D., Ph.D. and colleagues from the University of Lund, Sweden studied a population of 12,000 people. These people maintained their ancestral diet which was rich in coconuts and Coconut Oil.

- *Despite this population's Coconut Oil/high good fat diet, these researchers record having found NO evidence of heart disease at all. There was also no high blood pressure nor arteriosclerosis, no deaths from ischemic heart disease or from stroke, nor were there any such deaths in any medical records on this island.*

- *The results of this extensive study further revealed a "complete absence of diabetes, dementia and other degenerative diseases that were prevalent in the Western populations of the world."*

Even the elders of this culture, who lived up to 100 years of age, were still active and exhibited no signs of dementia or heart disease. This series of studies further confirmed the conclusion of many previous studies, which is:

- *Cultures whose diets were very high in good saturated fat from raw Coconut Oil were lean and strong, living long lives of exceptional health, free from Western diseases.*

(*...and you thought this Chapter was going to be just hocus pocus, didn't you?*)

Despite living on a *high good saturated fat diet*, consisting of between 45% and 60% fat from coconuts and raw Coconut Oil, all studied cultures *were lean and healthy.*
...Why ?
Because there is a critical difference between "good saturated fat" and "bad saturated fat." Coconut Oil/good saturated fat is life-giving, healing and strengthening to the body. It also provides a biological defense against a multitude of pathogens and diseases. Conversely, processed oils and hydrogenated oils have the *complete opposite effect* on your body, causing obesity, ill health and disease.

Give it to Me in a Nutshell (well, a Coconut Shell)...

Expansive research done on native cultures around the world has led to the following scientific conclusion and indisputable fact:

- *If Coconut Oil was an unhealthy fat (as many doctors today believe), then those populations which rely heavily on it as their daily staple would have surely died off centuries ago.*

- *Instead, these cultures have in fact prevailed and are thriving with excellent health and vitality, having a generational history of being virtually free from almost every western disease.*

Most Americans eat only 32-38 % fat in their daily diet, yet our country has one of the highest percentages of obesity and disease. *So why is our population fatter and sicker than those who eat twice as much saturated fat in their daily diets?*

The answer is simple: Because Western diets are strongly based upon unhealthy processed and hydrogenated oils. These processed oils have been proven to aggressively promote ill-health. Herein lies the critical difference:

- **It is NOT the AMOUNT of fat you eat that impacts your health;**
  It is the TYPE of fat you eat which causes sickness or health.
- **Raw Coconut Oil prevents weight gain, sickness and disease.**
  Processed Oils promote weight gain, sickness and disease.

- *You have just learned the most important facts in this chapter.*

3,000 Year Old Ayurvedic Medicine...

One of the best-known ancient protocols of healing is Ayurvedic Medicine. Coconut Oil has been used in Ayurvedic Medicine for healing and disease prevention for thousands of years, since the time of Sushruta Samhita. In both Ayurveda and Indian folk medicine, Coconut Oil is used to treat a wide variety of conditions such as burns, wounds, ulcers, skin fungus, kidney stones, choleric dysentery, epilepsy, heart disease, hepatitis C, psoriasis, eczema, fungal infections, parasites and atherosclerosis. Even today, a large percentage of the Eastern world still uses this ancient form of health care; because it works.

Today, in the country of India, Ayurvedic practitioners still provide healthcare to over 500 million people. For many years, Coconut Oil has also been used as the primary treatment in India for expelling parasites.

Dr. J.V. Hebbar teaches the following Ayurvedic uses for Coconut Oil:

> Nourishes undernourished body tissue
> Treats digestive and urinary disorders
> Treats diabetes
> Promotes hair quality & growth
> Alleviates eczema, psoriasis and other skin disorders
> Wound healing
> Normalizes respiratory rate in children with pneumonia
> (*Philippine Children's Medical Center study*)
> Reduce obesity

16

Simple Science Says...

A voluminous amount of compelling research has confirmed that the Medium Chain Fatty Acids (MCFA's) in Coconut Oil are antiviral, antibacterial, antifungal and antiparasitic and promote weight loss (...*what more can we ask for?*)

As we learned, *the MCFA Lauric Acid is Nature's most powerful antimicrobial. Raw, unrefined Coconut Oil is Nature's richest source of Lauric Acid.* One tablespoon of raw coconut oil has 7 grams of *Lauric Acid.* Additionally, Coconut Oil contains *Capric Acid*, and *Caprylic Acid* which also have very potent preventative and healing properties of their own.

Coconut Oil is also anti-inflammatory and aids in the absorption of Vitamins A, D, E and K. It strengthens the immune system and hormone production while supporting brain health, eye health and thyroid function. It has been proven effective in treating and preventing heart disease, blood clots, cancer, diabetes, hardening of the arteries, stroke, ulcers, Epilepsy and Alzheimer's.

Because of its unique health-giving properties, Coconut Oil has been used in IV's since World War II to revive critically ill patients. Because of its ability to build and strengthen the immune system, it was also a main ingredient in infant formulas. Even today, it is still a powerful remedy for malabsorption problems in infants and the elderly.

So Say the Experts...

Coconut Oil has also been shown to remedy systemic yeast infections. John P. Trowbridge, M.D., President of American College for the Advancement of Medicine and author of Book *The Yeast Syndrome* highly recommends

Caprylic Acid (found in Coconut Oil) to fight systemic candida yeast infections. This recommendation is confirmed by William Crook, M.D., a highly esteemed authority on yeast infections and author of *The Yeast Connection.* This is especially great news for patients who have adverse reactions to antibiotics or antifungal drugs. *It has been discovered that Caprylic Acid was equally effective against fungal infections as Nystatin,* the #1 antifungal prescription drug. Lastly, unlike most prescription drugs, Coconut Oil has no known negative side effects.

At this point, I hope you are getting very excited by the realization that this one simple addition to your daily diet can easily change your health, for the rest of your life
… you with me?

Let's Talk Antibiotics...
Standard medical protocol for a patient with any infection is to prescribe antibiotics. While this is sometimes effective, it usually comes with a price. Too many antibiotics in fact cause certain bacteria to become resistant, then requiring more and stronger drugs to fight them. Further, taking antibiotics too often or for too long will actually kill the "beneficial bacteria" in your gut, which is critical for your good health; as 70% of your immune system is in your gut. The good bacteria here are also needed to digest food, synthesize vitamins and to prevent the overgrowth of fungus or yeast cells in the body. This is why it is wise to take a probiotic whenever you're taking antibiotics. Probiotics support the good bacteria in your gut.

The Infection You Don't Know You Have...

Candida is a single-celled fungus or yeast cell which inhabits the intestinal tract. Taking antibiotics can kill off much of our good bacteria which then causes candida to grow in our bodies, unopposed. The harmful result is a systemic yeast infection caused by its overgrowth in the intestines. This kind of "silent" infection easily spreads through the entire body, usually going undetected for years. *The Fungal spores are so extremely minute that they don't show up on the average blood tests*. A specific test called "Chronic Fungal Fatigue Profile" performed on blood samples can indicate your level of systemic Candida infection. The symptoms include fatigue, poor digestion, brain fog, food sensitivities, weakened immune system, low mood, and joint pain. As you can see, these symptoms are so general they can be attributed to almost any ailment. So, *most people are not tested for Candida at all.* This is yet another compelling reason to eat Coconut Oil each day: to remedy a health disorder, to be proactive in preventing one…and to eradicate the systemic Candida that *you don't even know you have.*

Can Anything Kill a Virus…?

Funny you should ask. Viruses are generally impervious to all antibiotics. Although antibiotics are useful against some bacteria, *no antibiotic can kill a virus.* Drugs that purport to be "antiviral" may stop or slow down the spread of certain viruses, *but they are not able to kill or eliminate a virus*. Viruses can become deadly in people with depressed immune systems. This is why elderly people or those in poor health die from a simple flu virus each year.

Dr. Bruce Fife relays in his Book *The Coconut Oil Miracle* that he instructed one of his flu patients to take 3 tablespoons of raw unrefined Coconut Oil in lukewarm orange juice three times a day. The first day, symptoms got worse, as this was the body going through a *healing crisis*. The second day she felt better. All the symptoms were gone by day three.

Coconut Oil Kills Viruses...

As you now know, *the MCFA's in raw Coconut Oil literally rupture the outer cell wall of a virus or pathogen, causing their death.* This is what makes it a uniquely safe but powerful antibacterial, antiviral, antifungal and antiparasitic. The list of infections that Coconut Oil has been proven to successfully treat is amazing. They include Influenza, Herpes, and Measles, Mononucleosis, Hepatitis C, H. Pylori, Throat Infections, Pneumonia, Rheumatic Fever, Food Poisoning, Urinary Tract Infection, Meningitis, Gonorrhea, Toxic Shock Syndrome, Parasites and Fungal Infections such as a Yeast Infection, Candida and Thrush.

- Raw Coconut Oil is deadly to almost all microorganisms but is beneficial to the body.

Speaking of Breast Milk...

Mother's Breast Milk is the second highest natural source of MCFA's. It contains 6% germ-killing Lauric Acid. *Breast Milk is also a "Good Saturated Fat."* It is the Good Fat and the MCFA's in Breast Milk that have been proven to powerfully support and develop the brain, the eyes and the vulnerable immune system of infants. It also protects newborns from invading germs and infections while their fragile immune system is still developing (*because God knows what He's doing.*)

Dr. Mary Newport is a Neonatal Specialist, founding Director and Head of the newborn intensive care unit of

20

Spring Hill Regional Hospital in Florida. Dr. Newport affirms that because of its unique health-boosting properties, Coconut Oil is still used today to nurture and protect the underdeveloped immune systems of premature babies. Because it is so easily digested, hospitals also use it to treat malabsorption problems. As stated, it was used as a primary ingredient in infant formulas. Moreover, a nursing mother who consumes unrefined Coconut Oil will increase the level of MCFA's in her breast milk, providing the best possible protection and nutrition for her baby.

Dr. Jon J. Kabara, from Michigan State University, performed analytical studies on the Fatty Acids in raw Coconut Oil. He learned that the antimicrobial properties of its MCFA's become active when ingested. His research also confirmed the following MCFA's were present in Coconut Oil: *Caprylic Acid (C:8), Capric Acid (C:10), Myristic Acid (C:14), and Lauric Acid (C:12)*. Although all proved to have antimicrobial properties, he confirmed that *Lauric Acid* was the most powerful antimicrobial of them all. Raw Coconut Oil is composed of 48% Lauric Acid, 18% Myristic Acid, 7% Capric Acid, 8% Caprylic Acid, and 5% Caproic Acid.

- *Its 48% Lauric Acid content makes raw Coconut Oil the most powerful natural antimicrobial food ever known.*

- *Coconut Oil is all natural and has the added benefit of having no negative side effects or interaction with medications.*

Cell Permeability, What's That ...?

Our body is composed of approximately 37 Trillion cells. Each one of these cells has a cell wall made of what? *You guessed it...fat!* (*Look how smart you are.*) As we learned, our cells are like tiny *water balloons*, having a pliable soft, fatty outer membrane. This outer membrane must remain soft and permeable, meaning it allows things to pass through it easily so that oxygen and nutrients pass *into it* to feed the cell, and waste passes *out of it,* to keep the cell healthy. When the cell becomes sick or diseased, this outer wall of the cell becomes hard, like a piece of "M&M" candy, so that eventually, nothing can pass in or out of it. This is the beginning of disorders, disease and cell death. One of the many health benefits of Coconut Oil is that it keeps our 37 trillion cell walls *soft and permeable,* so there is *no interruption* with the minute by minute process of *"nutrients in"* and *"waste out."* This truth is both simple and hugely impactful, as the proper function of this vital process is the very foundation of our health.

How Diabetes Happens...

To run efficiently, every cell in our body commonly uses *glucose* as its food. Glucose requires insulin to enter the cell. Processed oils are very health-damaging fats. When eaten regularly, they disrupt the "insulin receptors" on your cell walls. This "locks the door" against receiving glucose from the food that we eat. As a result, the glucose builds up in the blood, creating Diabetes. What's worse is that the cell is then forced into starvation, becoming weak and stagnant. This is the recipe for cell death and disease.

Coconut Oil: Superfood for Each Cell ...

Processed, refined oils from the grocery store contain *long chain fatty acids.* Both glucose and long chain fatty acids *need insulin* to enter the cell to feed it. As stated, when insulin receptors are shut down or disrupted by bad fats, the cell can no longer receive glucose. Coconut Oil's MCFA's *have the ability to pass easily through the wall of sick or starving cells, feeding them without the need of insulin.*

Let's Read That Again…

- *The life-giving nutrients in raw Coconut Oil do NOT need insulin to get into your cells to feed them. Its healing MCFA's pass easily through the outer and the inner wall of every cell, to feed and heal the mitochondria (the cell's engine).*

- *So even when the insulin receptors on a sickly cell wall are shut down (as in diabetes), Coconut Oil is still able to get in to feed and resuscitate the dying cells.*

I am repeating the term "*MCFA's*" (medium chain fatty acids) as these are the key, active components abundant in Coconut Oil, which have profound healing and restorative effects on every cell in our body. I may also refer to them as *Good Fat.*

All Fats are NOT Created Equal…
You're gonna love this part.

When you eat processed oils, the body breaks them down into *little bundles of fat* and protein (lipoproteins). These little fat bundles are sent into the bloodstream where they are deposited into our fat cells. When physical activity demands it, fat from our fat cells is slowly removed and burned for fuel.

Now hear this…our body processes the good fat in raw Coconut Oil in a completely opposite manner. The fat in

23

Raw Coconut Oil is NOT packaged into little bundles of fat. (Can I get a Yay for that?)

Raw Coconut Oil does NOT circulate in the bloodstream like other fats; instead, *it travels to the liver where it is immediately converted into energy and a form of Cellular Superfuel called Ketones. Ketones are a high-octane fuel for the body and for the brain. Coconut Oil* does not raise blood sugar, so it is safe even for diabetics. Studies have shown it also reduces food cravings and hypoglycemia symptoms. With Coconut Oil, you don't have that empty hollow feeling you get when you eat a low-fat/no-fat diet.

The Short Version: Coconut Oil's Good Fat...
Satisfies hunger but does NOT store as fat
Converts to immediate energy
Feeds Ketone Superfuel to the brain
Revives sick and starving cells
Is Nature's most potent Antimicrobial
Boosts Immune System and Hormone production
Increases metabolism, and it tastes like butter
For many, it is seemingly a Miracle Food across the board.

- *"GOOD saturated fat" is in fact "GOOD for you."*

- *It is the TYPE of fat you eat which determines the condition of your health.*
Examples of good saturated fat are: Raw Coconut Oil, raw whole milk, real butter, avocado, salmon, mackerel, eggs, organ meats, red meats, dairy, raw nuts and breast milk.

Good Fat = a Smart, Healthy Child…

We learned how babies require good fat for their brains to grow properly and to develop their eyesight and immune system. Now you will learn that Good Fat is also critical for young, adolescent brains, *because their brains are still developing.*
(Lord knows, any parent of a teenager will agree their brain isn't fully developed!)

Good Fat in naturally fatty foods are crucial to adolescent brain development, eyesight and hormone production. Fatty fish, meats, eggs, raw whole milk, avocados, unrefined Coconut Oil, raw nuts, and raw milk are a healthy selection of good fats.

To restrict these good fats from a child's diet can prove detrimental to their physical and mental development. Sadly, many parents have resorted to feeding their children a breakfast consisting of skim milk and store-bought cereal containing processed grain, sugars and harmful processed vegetable oils. A much wiser choice would be a simple meal of oatmeal and blueberries with Coconut Oil in it, or eggs and toast with Coconut Oil or real butter on it. These much healthier choices would not only maintain their child's brain development, eye development and physical health but also protect against infections and illness. Dr. Johanna Budwig Ph.D. Biochemist and seven-time Nobel Prize Nominee discovered 60 years ago that *a growing child requires Good Fat to prevent hormonal deficiencies and behavioral problems.*

"Gimme the Skinny on Fat…"

Our energy-devouring brain requires both saturated and unsaturated fats to function, as well as for structural integrity and cell fluidity. By far, most of the fats that we eat go directly to be incorporated into the membranes of the cells that make up our brain and nervous system. Our nerve cell membranes are 50% fat, while the myelin sheath which protects the nerves is 70% fat.

- *The Body's daily demand for good fat is great and crucial.*

- *Our body is made up of trillions of cells with walls made of fat; the brain is 60% fat; the eyes are 40% fat; the body needs fat to manufacture hormones; the brain and eyes of children need fat to develop; the brain and the eyes of adults need fat to function properly. Now you have just learned why a "low-fat diet" is so detrimental to your hormones, your organs and your overall health.*

- *It is NOT the amount of fat you eat; it is the TYPE of fat you eat that makes you healthy or unhealthy (...this is a recording.)*

To deprive your body of Good Fat is the prelude to a lifetime of ill-health. Please don't let anyone talk you into a *"low fat/no fat"* diet for yourself or for your children. It is not only unsustainable, but grossly unhealthy, especially for developing children.

"What Happened in Alaska...?"

Founded in 1876, Johns Hopkins University is the oldest most respected research university in the country, and in the Western hemisphere. Johns Hopkins performed a unique study on the effect of dietary fat on our health. Step one, was to take a team of 30 scientists and run diagnostic

Mary Newport affirms she fed Coconut Oil to her husband several times a day to treat his advanced Alzheimer's condition. *Not only did it reverse his condition, but he lost 10 pounds, and his cholesterol and blood pressure were lowered.* (*Chapter 7, Alzheimer's*)

- *It has been well documented in numerous studies both in humans and animals that replacing processed vegetable oils and margarine with Coconut Oil resulted in reduction of stored fat.*

"How Do You Lose Weight on Coconut Oil...?"

So glad you asked. The superstar here would be the MCFA *Caprylic Acid*. Along with all its other health benefits, *Caprylic Acid* has a bonus effect of leaning down the body. *Caprylic Acid* and *Capric Acid* can also be found in MCT (medium chain triglycerides) oil. You may have heard of body builders taking MCT oil, *which is a concentrated form of 2 saturated fatty acids extracted from Coconut Oil.* MCFA's are efficiently turned into energy for the brain and body while also *promoting weight loss*. These good saturated fats in fact rev up their metabolism, helping these athletes plummet their BMI (Body Mass Index) down to its lowest level prior to competition.

Please note: Bodybuilders spend a great deal of time at the gym and on ultra rigid diets. So please don't be thinking you can run out and buy some MCT oil and become Mr. or Mrs. Olympia any time soon. The takeaway here is that, along with their rigid diets, bodybuilders eat a substantial amount of *Good Saturated Fat* derived from *Coconut Oil,* to lean down.

- MCT Oil is an extract of Coconut Oil and has *only 2 of its 5 MCFA's. It does NOT contain Lauric Acid*, which is the main healing ingredient in Coconut Oil. *In short, MCT oil can NOT kill microbes.*

- MCT Oil is *fractionated Coconut Oil*, which means it is *partially processed* via distillation and hydrolysis. *Therefore, the overall healthiest version of all 5 healing MCFA's in their natural state is raw unrefined Coconut Oil ...the Winner and still Champion.*

"Now Tell Us the Pig Story...!"

One fine day, the American Farmers Association decided to add Coconut Oil to their pigs' daily feed. They erroneously believed that, since Coconut Oil was a saturated fat, well then surely their pigs would gain weight and thereby bring them a better price per pig at market. However, what happened stunned everyone. *Not only did their pigs NOT gain weight; but in fact their pigs LOST weight!*

What happened here is that the unsuspecting farmers acted upon the *misinformation* that *all* saturated fat will make you gain weight. Now here is the best part. The quick-thinking farmers then *replaced the Coconut Oil with processed soybean oil.* When the *processed soybean oil* was added to the feed each day, what do you think happened? **The pigs gained all their weight back...plus MORE.**

Very happy for the Farmers. *Very sad for the pigs.*

Now I think I could safely say here that these pigs had not changed to a healthy diet, nor did they join the gym; but **these pigs LOST weight when Coconut Oil was added to their feed.** Period. This is one of my favorite stories,

30

because it is a crisp and alarmingly clear example of how profoundly Coconut Oil can work to lean down the body; and how frighteningly efficient processed oils are at causing weight gain.

The Big Takeaway here is:

- *When Coconut Oil was added to the Pigs' feed, they LOST WEIGHT.*

- *When the SAME AMOUNT of Soybean oil was added to their feed instead, the pigs REGAINED all the weight.*

- *Specifically, soybean oil contains Goitrogens, a chemical substance that disrupts the production of thyroid hormones. In short, it suppresses thyroid function. Hence, the pigs quickly regained their lost weight, and more.*

Now, you clearly understand the tremendous difference between Good Fat and Bad Fat.

"Dr. Sweeny Did What...?"

Way back in the 1920s, Dr. S. Sweeny had a peculiar practice of producing *reversible diabetes* in his first-year medical students. How did he produce diabetes in healthy young students? *He fed them a diet high in processed vegetable oil ...for only two days.*

This taught his students an invaluable lesson. The processed vegetable oil (Bad Fat) incorporated itself into the students' cell walls, *shutting down the cell wall's insulin receptors.* This prevented glucose from entering the cell. When the glucose (sugar) from food couldn't enter the cell, it then built up in their blood, *creating Diabetes*. This is an alarming example of how bad, processed oils can damage your health, in literally 2 days.

How did Dr. Sweeny then reverse his students' induced Diabetes? He healed their cell walls by simply eliminating all processed oils from their diet. By removing the root cause of their Diabetes, he *"plugged the holes in their boat."*

"What Did they Do to Pop…?"

In 2012, my father slipped and fell. He had to have a hip replacement and thereafter was sent to a rehabilitation center for physical therapy. Pop was 88 years old, in good health and he was on *NO medication* when he went into the Rehab.

But because of the grossly unhealthy diet he was being fed there, I am here to tell you, by day 3, that Rehab had Pop on *insulin injections for Diabetes. To clarify: Pop did NOT have Diabetes when he arrived.* It was a horror. My family and I were up in arms. As Dr. Sweeny had previously demonstrated, this was deeply disturbing proof of how a poor diet high in processed oils and unhealthy food can radically plummet someone's good health *in a matter of days*.

Needless to say, I demanded a conference call with the Director, the Head Nurse and the Chef to ascertain how they managed to turn my father into a Diabetic in 3 days. The Chef advised that he *cooks all his food with Soybean oil! Well, there you have it!* Like almost all processed oils, soybean oil disables the insulin receptors on the cell walls causing glucose to build up in the blood. The result is Diabetes. This was exactly like Dr. Sweeny's experiment, all over again.

I insisted that a specific and healthy diet be implemented for Pop immediately if not sooner. I had the nurses put notes on his food trays and on his door stating, *"NO PROCESSED OILS & NO WHITE CARBS FOR THIS PATIENT!"* I called every day to ask what he was eating *(oh yes they just loved me there.)* But guess what? Pursuant to this instruction, Pop's blood sugar dropped right back to normal. He was then taken off all insulin, *because the damaging cause had been removed.*

- *In just 2 days, Dr. Sweeny induced Diabetes in his young students by feeding them a diet high in processed vegetable oils. All cases of induced diabetes were completely reversed by removing the processed oils from their diet.*

- *In just 3 days, the Rehab induced diabetes in Pop by feeding him a diet high in processed vegetable oils and processed carbs. Pop's induced diabetes was completely reversed by removing all processed vegetable oils and processed carbs from his diet.*

Moral of the Story…
Slipping down the slope of ill-health can happen very quickly. But you can slam on the breaks by doing the following:

- *Replace all processed oils and fats in your kitchen with unrefined Coconut Oil.*

- *READ the LABEL on all packaged and bottled food items before you buy them. Refuse to buy or eat any food products with processed or hydrogenated oils in them, especially soybean or canola oil.*

"What About the Monkeys…?"

Compelling research has confirmed that Coconut Oil inhibits the action of carcinogenic agents which cause colon, skin, breast and other cancers in test animals.

It has been proven that when cancer is chemically induced in lab animals, *it is the TYPE of fat in their diet that determines the resulting number and size of cancerous tumors which develop*. *Processed polyunsaturated oils produced the most tumors and the largest tumors in laboratory animals injected with carcinogens. Monounsaturated fats (like Olive Oil) produced fewer tumors. But Coconut Oil produced the very least of all.*

When scientists attempted to induce cancer in lab monkeys, they discovered that by simply adding Coconut Oil to their food, *cancer development was often blocked*.
In many cases, Coconut Oil was proven to completely prevent tumor development in animals given very potent cancer-causing chemicals. This documented proof confirmed that raw unrefined Coconut Oil is in fact a very powerful anti-cancer food.
(Cohen & Thompson, 1987; Reddy, 1992.)

The Short Version…

- **Coconut Oil was shown to block cancer and tumor development in monkeys given cancer-causing chemicals.**
- **Processed polyunsaturated oils produced the most and the largest cancerous tumors in monkeys given cancer-causing chemicals.**

Regarding raw Coconut Oil vs processed vegetable oils, I tell my students this:

"If you remember nothing else I say, please just remember the stories about Dr. Sweeny, the Pigs and the Monkeys."

"Aren't all Fats the Same …?"
That would be a heck No.

As previously confirmed, most processed vegetable oils are known for their cancer-promoting effects, while Coconut Oil has been proven to substantially inhibit cancer and tumor growth. Processed oils attack the immune system and cause inflammation, while Coconut Oil strengthens the immune system and is anti-inflammatory; processed vegetable oils promote heart disease, weight gain and diabetes; Coconut Oil prevents and alleviates these conditions. In other words, *these 2 types of oils have a completely opposite effect on the body.* Coconut Oil is healing and strengthening, while the processed and hydrogenated oils induce weight gain, sickness and disease.

Processed Oils Greatly Suppress your Immune System…

It has been proven that processed vegetable oils *severely depress the immune system.* This alarming fact is so scientifically well known, that vegetable oil emulsions are given to patients who had organ transplants, *in order to intentionally suppress and disarm their immune system,* so that the donated (foreign) organ will be accepted by the patient's body.

I'm going to say this again:
- *Processed vegetable oils are so powerful in suppressing the immune system, that they are given to organ transplants patients, to avert rejection of their*

35

new organ. (This might be a good time to clean out your pantry.)

The majority of vegetable oils sold today are highly processed and refined. Not a health-giving thing. Chemical solvents are used to separate them from their source, then most of these oils are boiled, bleached and deodorized, being heated to temperatures around 400 degrees Fahrenheit. Finally, chemical preservatives are usually added. Is this the kind of franken-food you wish to eat and feed to your family?

Be aware that the insidious results of using these processed oils in your cooking, coupled with the fact that they are also in most of the packaged food you buy, ensure you are *unconsciously eating a steady diet* of sickness-promoting factors. The negative effects of this are not immediately visible, but progress silently and harmfully, building up in your body over months and years, undermining your health.

Processed Polyunsaturated Oils are Chemically Unstable...
Jurg Loliger, Ph.D., of Nestle Research Center in Switzerland, advises in his book *Free Radicals & Food Additives* that *processed polyunsaturated oils have a very high probability of going rancid due to their chemical instability.* When exposed to heat, sunlight or artificial light, the rancidity expedites. *His conclusion was that many of the processed vegetable oils you buy from the store are already at least partially rancid. Dr. Loliger asserts that a processed vegetable oil may be very rancid while not giving any indication of this by way of taste or smell. He further asserts that saturated fats are much more stable.* They can be

exposed to heat, light and oxygen without forming any discernible degree of rancidity or free radical formation. Most saturated fats remain stable even when used for cooking.

Tropical Oils were widely used as a Preservative in many of our Foods up until the late 1980s.

As a result, these foods remained fresher for longer periods of time and were better for your health. Coconut Oil is highly stable and does not go quickly rancid, as the unstable polyunsaturated processed oils do. Almost all packaged and processed foods now contain health-damaging, highly processed vegetable oils. In 1990, the fast food industry abandoned the use of more stable good fats like natural beef tallow and began using processed vegetable oil to cook their french fries. *This doubled the fat content of their fries and also replaced Good Fat with Bad Fat.* The choice of using processed vegetable oils (especially soybean oil) is so much unhealthier because it contains toxic trans fatty acids. As a result, fast foods started having a radical effect on the rise of blood cholesterol, obesity and heart disease in the U.S. population.

Fast Food, Slow Death…

Around 1990, one of the biggest fast-food chains in the world switched from cooking with beef tallow (all natural) to processed vegetable oils. By 2002, this chain was using a processed *soybean-corn* blend. *Double whammy.* The health consequences of this were so egregious that they spawned an eye-opening documentary and *social experiment* called *Super-Size Me.* Through the valiant efforts of Dr. Morgan Spurlock, this experiment shouted a message loud and clear about the severe health consequences of eating fast food (bad fats). Begun in 2002, his experiment documents in great detail just how powerfully and how quickly bad cholesterol and unhealthy processed oils destroy the human body.

Dr. Spurlock committed to eating fast food from a popular fast-food chain 3 times a day for 30 days. Week by week he became fatter and sicker. Here are the results he and his doctors documented:

- Day 5, he gained 10 pounds
- Day 7, pressure in chest
- Day 9, depressed for no reason
- Day 10, blood pressure has spiked
- Day 17, decreased sex drive; blood pressure up, 150/90 cholesterol rose over 200
- In 18 days, his liver was inflamed and was reducing in size.
  By this time, he had consumed 12 pounds of bad fat and bad cholesterol.
- Next he developed a liver disease called NASH (non-alcoholic steatohepatitis).
- Day 30: His weight increased by 25 pounds. His cholesterol shot up 65 points.
- He was depressed and exhausted. He had no sex drive. *He had doubled his chances of coronary heart disease. He almost doubled his risk for stroke, heart attack, heart failure, liver disease and organ failure.*

Dr. Spurlock's results were measured, confirmed and documented by 3 doctors including a Cardiologist, a Nutritionist and a Physiologist. Ultimately, his doctors warned him to stop this experiment because *he was in danger of total organ failure.*

Released in 2004, Dr. Spurlock's Documentary *Super-Size Me* was indeed a wake-up call. When Scientists publish report after report about how *bad oils* damage your body, most people don't hear or don't care; but if you watch just *one movie* showing the same results happening to a real live person, *well now, we are all standing at attention aren't we?* Dr. Spurlock risked his own health by eating an exceedingly unhealthy diet, allowing his body to be damaged for 30 days to a nearly fatal state. But he successfully proved to the American public how powerfully these bad fats and fast-food meals undermine our health.

The Short Version…

- *In just 30 days, a diet high in processed polyunsaturated oils, bad cholesterol and highly processed foods caused a 25-pound weight gain, blood pressure and cholesterol to shoot up…and organ functions to SHUT DOWN.*

- *While heart, liver and kidney functions plummeted, the risk of heart disease, heart failure, kidney failure and liver failure had DOUBLED.*

Understandably, none of us are eating 3 meals a day of fast-food (I hope), but do take an inventory of how many times a week or a month you are eating it. When you're pressed for time, do you stop at a fast-food place for yourself or for your kids because you are in a rush? Now that you know what you know, please reconsider. Because the negative impact of these "every now and then" toxic meals are adding up inside your bodies, in slow motion.

How Did the U.S. Population Get FAT…?

Disturbingly, the American diet lost the war between the use of *healthy Topical Oils vs processed soybean oil.*

Soybean Lobbyists successfully convinced America that highly processed soybean oil was healthier than previously used natural oils like Coconut Oil and beef tallow. Even movie theaters began using health damaging processed soybean oil to make their popcorn. The American Soybean Association emerged victorious in their widespread propaganda that soybean oil (highly processed polyunsaturated oil) was healthier than all natural good saturated tropical fats. Soybean oil has become ubiquitous (it's everywhere) in the American diet. Next time you go food shopping, *please read the labels.* You will be shocked to find how many packaged products have soybean oil in their top 5 ingredients. Soybean oil and/or hydrogenated soybean oil is now in most salad dressings, cereal, crackers, chips, cookies, cupcakes, and peanut butter. In addition to being in a vast amount of packaged and processed foods, it is usually the main ingredient in almost all margarines and butter substitutes. Two-thirds of the vegetable oils sold in America today comes from soybean oil, containing up to *50% trans fatty acids, a very bad fat.*

In 1982, an average restaurant meal contained approximately 2.4 grams of trans fat. By 2013, *that same meal* contained *19.2 grams of trans fat (9x more)*, simply because they *changed the type of oil in their kitchen.* It is no wonder that in this country there has been such a marked increase in heart disease, stroke, cancer, diabetes, arteriosclerosis, obesity and since 1982. These statistics are the alarming result of the misinformation about healthy tropical plant fats coupled with the push for the use of unhealthy processed soybean oil. It was a tug of war between scientific evidence and political propaganda, wherein, sadly the soybean propaganda has won.

Simple Science Says…

Hundreds of scientific reports conclude it is the overconsumption of processed vegetable oils in processed foods that have grossly contributed to the obesity and overall poor health of most western civilizations.

Saturated fats are classified as long chain fatty acids (LCFA's), short chain fatty acids and medium chain fatty acids (MCFA's). Each of these groups has a markedly different biological effect on the body, confirms Mary Enig, Ph.D. Biochemist and Lipid Expert. Dr. Enig attests that lab *animals fed hydrogenated oils (trans fat) were no longer able to properly utilize insulin*. Her research further documents that Trans Fatty Acids/Trans Fats proved to have the most damaging impact on health. Dr. Enig confirms:

- *It is the processed vegetable oils and Trans Fats that are proven to be the predominant cause of heart disease, MS, cancer, diabetes, diverticulitis, arteriosclerosis and a host of other systemic disorders.*

MCFA's in Coconut Oil have the unique ability to penetrate through both the outer and the inner cell wall of sick or dying cells to feed and to resuscitate them. Whereas, soybean, canola and other processed vegetable oils *have the exact opposite effect*. They shut down the insulin receptors on the cell walls, thereby preventing food (glucose) from passing from the bloodstream into the cell. This action triggers a host of health problems.

- *Processed oils and hydrogenated oils promote and sustain ill health.*

41

- *They suppress the immune system, making you more vulnerable to infection, disease and weight gain..*

- *Specifically, Soybean Oil contains Goitrogens, an anti-thyroid chemical, which suppresses thyroid function,* decreases metabolism and causes weight gain. This is exactly what happened to the pigs when farmers added soybean oil to their feed.

"Why Do I Care about Hydrogenated Oils…?"
What is the unhealthiest form of processed oil?

A *hydrogenated* one.

Hydrogenated oils are very highly processed so that they become artificially solid at room temperature, like Crisco, margarine and some brands of peanut butter. Hydrogenation is a chemical process whereby the oil is heated up to 400 degrees and then bombarded with hydrogen molecules. *Yumm.*

This process causes the oil to contain *trans-fatty acids* which Dr. Enig confirms are the most destructive to your health. Hydrogenation is widely used to make margarine and shortening. These products are up to *40% trans-fat.* Most processed vegetable oils contain up to *20% trans-fat.* Hydrogenated oils are also found in many prepackaged foods, (e.g., peanut butter, corn chips, cookies) and should be clearly listed on the product label under "Ingredients."

- *Many Lipid Experts agree that hydrogenated/trans-fat has the greatest impact on cardiovascular disease than any other fat.*

- *You don't have to be a Scientist to simply read the label to see if there is any weight-gaining, disease-*

causing processed oil or hydrogenated oil in the ingredients of the food you are about to buy.

"What About Those Nurses…?"

A report in the New England Journal of Medicine on November 20, 1997 documents a 14 year study performed on 80,000 nurses. Only those nurses who had the largest amount of *trans fat* in their diet developed a *53% higher probability of having a heart attack or stroke*, compared to the study group who ate little or no trans-fat. *Amazingly,* **the results showed it did not matter how much fat these women ate, but only what kind of fat they ate.** *(Where have we heard that before?)*

This discovery was confirmed by the Harvard School of Public Health and Brigham Women's Hospital in Boston. It has been well documented by *hundreds of studies that there is a drastic difference between "good saturated fat" and "bad saturated fat."* Yet many doctors today continue to warn their patients against eating *any* saturated fats at all, as if they are all the same.

"How Do I Know If I'm Eating Trans-Fat…?"

If you're eating margarine, shortening or ANY product that has hydrogenated or partially hydrogenated oil in it…you are eating bad trans fat. Just read the label.

Fun Fact:

The difference between Fats and Oils is:
"Fats" naturally take solid form at room temperature.
"Oils" naturally take liquid form at room temperature.

Good Fat Burns Fat…
Coconut Oil Speeds up Metabolism (Thermogenesis)…

Thermogenesis is the stimulation of cellular activity. When we eat foods that *increase thermogenesis* we are also *increasing our metabolism* and firing up our fat burning furnace. Protein-rich foods such as meat also increase thermogenesis. This is why high protein/high fat diets trigger weight loss by increasing metabolism.

Science has proven that raw Coconut Oil can speed up your metabolism more than protein. Confirmed in his Book *The Coconut Oil Miracle* Dr. Bruce Fife attests, *"The MCFA's (Good Fats) in Coconut Oil shift the body's metabolism into a higher gear, so you burn more calories. Because the MCFA's increase the metabolic rate, Coconut Oil is a dietary fat that can actually promote weight loss!"* (Fife, 2013*)*

- *The LCFA's (Long Chain Fatty Acids) in processed and hydrogenated oils are stored as fat.*

- *The MCFA's (Medium Chain Fatty Acids) in Coconut Oil are NOT stored as fat; instead, they are easily and rapidly burned for energy.*

This is why so many people lose weight as a delightful side effect of switching from processed vegetable oils to eating raw unrefined Coconut Oil. World renowned authority on Nutrition, Dr. Julian Whitaker confirms: *"LCFA's are like heavy wet logs you put on a campfire. MCFA's are like rolled up newspaper soaked in gasoline. They not only burn brightly, but burn up the wet log as well."* (Murray, 1996)

- *Research findings support Dr. Whitaker's belief, demonstrating that MCFA's eaten over six days increased fat burning by an amazing 50%.*

Supporting research findings confirm test subjects who were fed MCFA's had an increase in their energy expenditure (calorie burning) *of 48% higher than normal.*

This energy expenditure increased by 65% in obese test subjects. Results showed that eating MCFA's at a single meal keeps metabolism elevated for 24 hours. Additional studies confirm that over a 6-hour period, *the thermogenic, calorie-burning effect of MCFA's in Coconut Oil was three times greater than that of the LCFA's in processed polyunsaturated vegetable oils.*

Research performed at McGill University in Canada affirmed:

- *By removing all processed oils (LCFA's) from your daily diet and replacing them with MCFA's (raw Coconut Oil), you can lose up to 36 pounds in a year.*

How Processed Oils Make You Fat...

Polyunsaturated oils depress thyroid activity, thereby lowering your metabolic rate, inducing weight gain. Coconut Oil does exactly the opposite by increasing metabolic rate, inducing weight loss. It has been proven that processed polyunsaturated oils, like soybean oil, promote weight gain more than any other type of oil, including lard and beef tallow.

Ray Peat, Ph.D. is an endocrinologist who specializes in the study of hormones. Dr. Peat confirms that *polyunsaturated oils block thyroid hormone secretion and the response of our tissues to this hormone.* As a result, our metabolism dramatically slows down because we become deficient in thyroid hormones, causing weight gain. In effect, processed oils and fats *assault the thyroid causing it to weaken and malfunction.* This results in weight gain and many other health consequences.

Just Remember those Pigs…
- *They lost weight when the farmers added Coconut Oil to their feed.*
- *They gained that weight back and more when Soybean oil was added to their feed, instead.*

Why…?

Because the "anti-thyroid" chemical (Goitrogens) in soybean oil is alarmingly effective at suppressing the thyroid which, in turn, lowers metabolic rate, causing weight gain. *The pigs ate the same food, yet they suddenly gained weight…sound familiar ?*

Forget the Experts. What Say the Teenagers…?
A Good Quality Raw Coconut Oil "Tastes Like Butter."

One fine day, my teenage son and his four friends were rabble rousing in my kitchen, when I took out my jar of Coconut Oil. In accordance with Teenage Know-it-All fashion, they quickly and enthusiastically pooh-poohed my precious Coconut Oil.

They threw down the gauntlet.

I did the only thing a Mother can do…I challenged them to a taste test. The stakes were high: if they thought my Coconut Oil tastes like Butter, then they have to eat it from this day forward without complaint. But, if they could tell the difference between the taste of Butter and the taste of Coconut Oil, then I would banish Coconut Oil from our kitchen forever. *Ohh Yes, it was a bold wager; but I was that sure of the outcome.*

So then gathered the arrogant albeit somewhat lovable teenagers at my kitchen counter, their mouths watering as the aroma of the raisin toast I was making taunted them. I laid down the rules. For them to be victorious, they had to be able to tell the difference between the taste of melted butter and melted Coconut Oil on the raisin toast, that is, they had to perceive which was which.

Please note:

Both butter and Coconut Oil are clear when melted so they look the same on hot toast. Also, a good quality Coconut Oil even smells the same as butter.

The stage was set. I made 6 pieces of raisin toast, cutting them in half and putting undisclosed toppings on them. I gave the boys sampling number 1, waited til they gobbled it up, then served them sampling #2. The results came in fast and furious.

My son shouted in triumph, *"MOM!...the first batch was definitely the butter and the 2nd batch was the Coconut Oil!"*

A sly smile spread slowly across my face as I smugly advised, *"Lovey...they were ALL Coconut Oil."*

(...and that's why I'm the Big Dog...;)

TESTIMONIALS (everyone's favorite part)...
Strep Throat Cured / Prevented...

I suffered from severe bouts of strep throat most of my life, since I was about 7 years old. This included a very high fever, swollen throat glands, constricted breathing and horrible pain in my throat. This afflicted me at least four times a year. No amount of any antibiotic did a thing, as the *streptococcus bacteria* would ravage my weary body for 10 days to 2 weeks each and every time.

The frightening thing was that I wasn't "catching" *Strep throat* from anyone. I realized the *Strep bacteria was happily living inside my body* and just emerging whenever I got run down. All antibiotics were powerless against my resistant Strep and only served to kill off my good bacteria, making me weak and causing yeast infections. Then one day I learned about the miraculous healing properties of unrefined Coconut Oil. Could it be that this delicious food could rid me of this lifelong plague?

...I was all ears and all in.

The first most remarkable thing I discovered was that a high-quality unrefined Coconut Oil actually did taste very much like butter! Good thing, because I was absolutely *not* a fan of the taste of processed coconut. I began cooking with only raw Coconut Oil every day and eating it several times a day. I put it in my hot tea, on my toast, on all my vegetables, in my oatmeal and in my protein and fruit smoothies. The taste was undetectable in the smoothies, but everywhere else it added a rich, buttery flavor and creamy texture. I loved it.

Did it work...?

To this day, 12 years later, I have never had even one more strep throat attack.

...Not one.

The Coconut Oil successfully exterminated the latent resistant strep bacteria that had been living in my body for decades.

Oh yesss, I became a believer at warp speed. I replaced every single oil and fat in my kitchen with unrefined Coconut Oil. I cooked with it, making healthy fried eggs, or sauteing garlic and onions for my favorite Italian dishes, using it when reheating veggies or pasta leftovers. It consistently added its buttery flavor wherever I used it.

48

Coconut Oil was officially my favorite health maintenance food…*and my new best friend.*

Mother, 90 Years Old
Alzheimer's Symptoms Reversed…

Years ago, my mother was diagnosed with Alzheimer's Disease. It was just heartbreaking to see my mother fading away from reality, not even remembering family members or the names of her own children. She didn't know where she was. Finding her way to her bedroom was an impossibility. She no longer remembered what a refrigerator was. Even though she was 90 years old, each day she would ask me to call her mother, who had been dead for 40 years. Although we flew across the country to get to my house, she had no recollection of even being on a plane. She was a frail 95 pounds and just a shell of the Mother I knew. Her eyes had a distant glaze over them, confirming that there was only a hazy connection between her mind and the outside world. Mother was detached and disengaged. She was unplugged from life.

…and I wasn't having any of it.

I dove into my treasure chest of healing to collect everything that would restore her physical and mental health. I discovered a book called *Alzheimer's Disease, What If There Was a Cure?* by Dr. Mary Newport. In her book, Dr. Newport documented in great detail how *she reversed her husband's severe Alzheimer's by feeding him Coconut Oil.*
I was on it.

I began feeding my mother 8 Tablespoons of Coconut Oil a day, in her oatmeal, in her tea, on her vegetables, in soup, on potatoes, on toast, in protein smoothies. The changes in mother were dramatic. In 2 weeks, there was a striking improvement in her perception of the world around her and in her spirit and vibrancy. One day she just looked at me and said, "My mom is dead isn't she?" I replied "Yes, Mother. You're 90 years old now." She understood. She reasoned that if she is 90, then her mother cannot still be alive. Mother was now looking at me with clarity. The fog had lifted from her mind. *The lights came on in her eyes.*

I know that no Author should be throwing the word "Miracle" around, but I have to tell you…it sure felt like a Miracle to me.

Mother continued to improve daily, becoming very comfortable and familiar with her surroundings. After 4 months, my niece was getting married back in Pennsylvania. This meant another cross-country trip with mother. But what a different trip this was. Mother was fully engaged, helping me pack and choosing her dress for the wedding. On the plane she chatted with other passengers and enjoyed the flight.

At the wedding, mother actually recognized people. Her eyes were clear and bright. She was *engaged and present.* She was no longer trapped inside her own mind. She was enjoying normal conversations, making jokes and was just *alive again.* My mother was back, released from the prison of her mind. I was thrilled and thankful. Our relatives were just amazed at the transformation. It sure seemed like a Miracle to them too.

I keep 2 favorite photos of my mother from that time. Photo #1 was when she first came to live with me. Her skin was dull and sallow, her eyes were sunken and blank. She was emotionless and disconnected. Photo #2 was taken 4 months later at the wedding. In this second photo mother's skin is pink, her eyes bright and joy is shining from her face. And yes, you can clearly see *the lights are on in her eyes.*

In Chapter 7, I will go into much more detail on how Coconut Oil reverses/reduces Alzheimer's symptoms. For now, let me just remind you that raw Coconut Oil is NOT processed by the body as other fats. **Coconut Oil is taken up by the liver and converted into Ketones. Ketones are a high-octane fuel that is immediately delivered to the brain. This results in the powerful resuscitation of starving and dying brain cells.**

I am confirming to you that my mother was living, breathing proof that this is true.

Parkinson's Symptoms Reversed...

Helen was a student in my Wellness Class. She advised that her husband was suffering from Parkinson's Disease at the young age of 49. He was a very large man, Over 6 feet tall. His condition was deteriorating. At this point in time, he was stumbling and sometimes falling down when he walked and could no longer climb the stairs properly. I gave my initial instructions, loud and clear, as follows:

1) *THROW OUT ALL processed oils and fats from your kitchen.*
2) *Eat 6-8 Tablespoons of Raw Coconut Oil every day.*
3) *Use ONLY raw unrefined Coconut Oil for cooking, for everything.*

Helen's husband diligently complied with these simple but life-changing instructions. He cooked with only raw Coconut Oil and added several tablespoons to the protein smoothies he drank every day. His health visibly improved within the first 2 weeks. By week 4, he had regained his balance and strength. By week 6, he went back to exercising and was able to return to work. He thanked me personally for his seemingly miraculous recovery. (But we know it wasn't really me that healed him ;)

This is an exciting example of how the simple choice of eating a simple food most likely prevented this good man from ending up in a wheelchair. He regained his balance, his good health and his life, by just *Following the Recipe:*

- *He "Plugged the holes in his Boat" by throwing out all processed oils.*
- *He "Followed the Recipe" by REPLACING those bad oils with unrefined Coconut Oil.*

Two simple, but life-changing changes. The Power of Choice.

Helicobactor Pylori Bacteria Killed...

H. Pylori can be picked up through contaminated food or water. It is a highly resistant bacteria which infects and inflames the lining of the stomach. The Mayo Clinic attests that this bacteria is the primary cause of peptic stomach ulcers and that more than 50% of the world's population has some level of it in their stomach. Because it is antibiotic-resistant, the Mayo Clinic confirms that an H. Pylori stomach infection *"can last a lifetime."* (Mayo Clinic, 2022)

Ron, a close friend of mine, had been battling this stomach ailment for over 10 years. He suffered from pain and burning caused by this resistant bacteria. Ron was put on oral antibiotics for weeks and months, with no success. He was even hospitalized and given very strong IV antibiotics, to no avail. The overuse of these antibiotics only served to weaken his immune system and exhaust his body, but had no effect on the *H. Pylori.*

One day, while listening to his tale of woe, I realized I had just recently learned 2 very important facts in this regard:

1. 90% of all stomach ulcers are caused by the *H. Pylori* bacterium.
2. Coconut Oil *has been shown to kill the H. Pylori* Bacterium.

I proceeded to share my newfound knowledge with Ron, instructing him to put 5-8 tablespoons of unrefined Coconut Oil into his food or smoothies each day. This is such a simple yet powerful thing to add to your daily diet, as a good quality virgin unrefined Coconut Oil melts easily into hot foods and also blends very well into cold smoothies. My friend followed my advice.

It took only 3 weeks of eating Coconut Oil to rid him of the stomach pain he had suffered for 10 years. Simply eating unrefined Coconut Oil every day *eliminated all traces and symptoms of the H. Pylori bacteria; and it never returned.*

- *He also lost 6 pounds.*

John, 43 Years Old
Rhabdomyolysis, Rare Muscle Disease Healed…

In 2017, a woman named Claudia came into my Health and Wellness Class. Claudia was distraught, advising that her husband had a rare muscle disease called *Rhabdomyolysis.* This is a disease that causes muscle tissue breakdown and the release of a damaging protein into the blood which ultimately causes kidney damage. The Doctors advised *there was no hope of cure.*

John was given 5 prescriptions, including a muscle relaxer, antidepressant, sleeping pill, blood pressure medicine and painkillers. As a result, this poor man's condition only worsened. He couldn't walk even short distances without being in severe pain and needing to be on oxygen.

Sadly, John lost his job of 17 years and ended up depressed and in a wheelchair at the young age of 43 years old. Claudia advised he had been depressed, out of work and on Disability for the past three years.

After much prayer and heartache, Claudia confessed she joined my class as a last-minute hope. She was desperate to find a solution for her husband and for the hugely negative impact his poor health has had on their young family.

At this juncture, let me share the most beautiful thing about using Coconut Oil to treat a disorder: Even if you don't know exactly what is wrong with the Patient, having them eat *raw Coconut Oil should at the very least, improve the symptoms and, more often than not, it also eradicates the cause.* Coconut Oil has never been found to worsen any condition or cause harm. *This fact is a timeless Gem of Wisdom that you should tuck inside your Wellness Toolbox. Pursuant to this knowledge, I was undeterred by this man's "incurable" diagnosis.*

.

I delivered my unwavering instructions:
1. THROW OUT ALL PROCESSED FATS AND OILS from your kitchen.
2. Eat 8 Tablespoons of unrefined Coconut Oil per day, every day.
3. Use ONLY unrefined Coconut Oil for cooking, for everything.
4. Do *Oil Pulling* 20 minutes every day (*Chapter 4*).

5. Take 5 drops of Cellfood in water 2x a day
(Cellfood, *Chapter10*).

I also instructed that John drink 2 raw fruit smoothies per day with raw Coconut Oil and with 20 grams of protein (from protein powder). Because I knew his muscles needed protein for regeneration and repair.

Each week in class, Claudia reported that John was rigidly following my instructions as he was very desperate to regain his life.

In just THREE WEEKS, Claudia ran into my classroom in tears, revealing that her husband had just taken their 4 children to the Zoo. She affirmed he walked around at the Zoo for 2 hours without needing oxygen, painkillers…or his wheelchair! He was also off his blood pressure medication and antidepressants. What a Victory! Claudia and her husband were elated, and, oh so was I.

Claudia later confirmed that after 6 weeks, John was off all 5 of his medications and he had abandoned his wheelchair completely.

Simple choices made radical changes in John's life and the life of his family. He went from being diagnosed as "incurable" to resurrecting his health and his quality of life, in just 6 weeks. He "Followed the Recipe."

Yep, Coconut Oil.

Restored Eyesight, Diabetes Reversed…

Karl was a 60-year-old man diagnosed with Diabetes. He was put on a prescription medication called Atorvastatin. To his horror, he found that this medication was causing him *to progressively lose his eyesight. Karl affirmed that after only two weeks on this medication, he was unable to see his feet when he looked down!* Due to this alarming side effect, he stopped taking this medication.

I instructed him to eliminate all processed oils from his diet and begin taking 5-8 Tablespoons of Coconut oil every. I also asked him to take 7 drops of Cellfood each day (Chapter 10).

Day by day, Karl's eyesight steadily improved. *After only 2 weeks, he affirmed he was able to see his feet again! After 6 weeks, his blood tests came back "normal."*

This blood test confirmed that his blood sugar and bad cholesterol went down to HALF of their original levels!

We were both so thrilled!

Knowledge truly is Power.

Skin Lesion Disappeared...

Some years ago, I contracted some kind of lesion on my thigh, perhaps from the gym. It was raised, bumpy and alarming. I tried everything on it, but it persisted. Finally, I thought, let me just rub some raw Coconut Oil on it. To my great surprise, it disappeared completely in 2 days.

I had no idea then what that growth was on my leg was, nor do I know even now. But 2 things I do know: The raw Coconut Oil made it disappear in 2 days, and it never returned.

Stye in the Eye Healed...

We used raw unrefined Coconut Oil on my son to heal his infected tear duct (stye) in his eye. I gently rubbed a small amount of the Coconut Oil over the entire eye, 3 times a day. His eye was healed by day 3. Coconut Oil safely kills most pathogens while gently nourishing and lubricating the eye.

Acne Relieved ...

My friend Sarina's son had a severe case of acne. Acne is caused by acnes bacteria, which is one of the many bacteria that Coconut Oil kills. I had her son eat unrefined Coconut Oil several times a day. Further, I asked him to mix the Coconut Oil with a drop of Essential Oil of Eucalyptus and apply it to the affected area twice a day.

In one week, he showed great improvement in his skin; after 5 weeks his symptoms were almost completely gone.*

- *Please note: To achieve these remarkable results, I also instructed that he eliminate all unhealthy fats, fried food, fast foods and corn from his diet.*

Weight Loss / Fitness...

My cousin Janet had a very successful bodybuilding career, even achieving the Title of Miss World. She advised that while she was in training, she ate several Tablespoons of MCT *at each meal*. MCT oil is Caprylic Acid and Capric Acid extracted from Coconut Oil. To be clear, she ate many tablespoons per day of *Good Saturated Fat* (MCFA's) to achieve her *astounding low 9% body fat*.

Of course, Janet ate a religiously healthy diet and trained professionally at the gym for long hours each and every day. The point being made here is that she ingested a great deal of *"Good Fat"* to rev up her metabolism and to lean down to her lowest possible BMI (body mass index). Janet is 70 years old today and is a Professional Trainer. She is 105 pounds and *she still looks flipping awesome.*

Please remember:

Coconut Oil has the highest amount of germ-killing Lauric Acid; whereas, MCT oil has none.

Excerpts of Testimonials:
Dr. Bruce Fife, The Coconut Oil Miracle (2013)…

Weight Loss…

Dr. Bruce Fife advised that he tried everything to lose weight: eating margarine, vegetable oils, low fat/no fat diets to no avail. *It wasn't until he replaced all his kitchen fats with Coconut Oil that he lost 20 pounds.* He finally realized *he was eating the wrong kind of oils*. Dr. Fife attests that when he replaced processed oils with Coconut Oil, he lost 20 pounds in a matter of months without dieting, and the weight stayed off.

Weight Loss…

After decades of being overweight, Sharon was depressed and discouraged. She was faithfully eating processed polyunsaturated fats, erroneously believing this would help her; but it only caused her to continue to gain weight. After reading Dr. Fife's book, she *decided to abandon all polyunsaturated and hydrogenated oils, and switch instead to raw Coconut Oil.*

The results amazed her. She affirms she lost 20 pounds in a matter of weeks without changing anything else in her diet. After one year, the weight has stayed off. Sharon concludes by stating that she was *convinced that it was the processed polyunsaturated oils that made her gain weight, and it was the Coconut Oil that helped her lose it.*

Dandruff Relief…

Dr. Bruce Fife advises he had suffered from severe dandruff since he was a teenager. Medicated shampoos had limited effect but never eradicated the dandruff or the cause.

Dandruff is caused by a fungus (*Malassezia*). After learning that Coconut Oil kills fungus, he decided to massage some Coconut Oil in his hair and on his scalp. Dr. Fife explains his remarkable results as follows:

"The result was phenomenal. After a single application all the dandruff was gone. I couldn't believe it was that easy. Coconut Oil is now a regular part of my personal hair care regimen." (Fife, 2013)

Psoriasis...

A patient who suffered from severe psoriasis on his face and chest most of his adult life was at his wit's end. Nothing worked for this patient. Every few days, his condition would flare up and skin would become so bad it would crack and bleed. Several doctors advised there was nothing they could do to help him. He started eating Coconut Oil which improved his condition but it did not go away completely, until he decided *to apply* Coconut Oil to the affected areas. He was overjoyed to see immediate improvement the very next day. He continued applying the Coconut Oil to his face and chest each day. To his amazement, within a few days the skin on his face and neck which was previously *dry and leathery* had now become soft and smooth. He no longer had inflammation or scaling.

He declared it was the best his skin has looked in 20 years.

Plantar Warts Healed...

Coconut Oil is a perfect base for making herbal ointments and salves. An example is a potent salve called *"GOOT"* (*garlic oil ointment*) made up of crushed raw garlic and raw Coconut Oil. Mark Conlee, the Editor of *Positive Health Magazine*, advised he is always amazed at what this ointment can accomplish. He prescribed it for a patient named Dan, who had a severe case of plantar warts and athlete's foot, *the worst he had ever seen. Plantar warts are caused by a virus; Athletes' feet are caused by fungus. Fortunately, Coconut Oil kills both.* Mark made some *GOOT* and told Dan to apply it to his feet everyday.

Two weeks later, he met with Dan again. Mark confirmed that *Dan took off his socks to reveal what looked like a new set of feet!* He called it a *magical transformation as both the fungal infection and the plantar warts had completely disappeared.* Dan confirmed that after 10 days of using the garlic and Coconut Oil mixture, the plantar warts just peeled off.

Sunburn Pain / Reduced Skin Inflammation...

Dr. Bruce Fife advised he used Coconut Oil one day on a bad sunburn. He affirmed his sunburn pain was gone in about thirty minutes. He also witnessed Coconut Oil relieved his patient's chronic skin inflammation within days. This caused him to uncover the research of Dr. S. Sadeghi, et al, which revealed that "Coconut Oil reduces proinflammatory chemicals in the body."

Fun Fact:
- *Coconut Oil was a common ingredient in many of the first commercially produced sunscreens and suntan lotions; but now it has been generally replaced by chemicals.*

Boost Immune System, Boost Thyroid / Weight Loss...

Registered Nurse Marie, advises she uses virgin Coconut Oil as a foundational product for all her clients. After 30 years in the world of healing, she asserts that *Coconut Oil is one of the most powerful modalities she has ever worked with.*

Marie confirms that her patients start with 3 to 4 Tablespoons a day of unrefined Coconut Oil because it works well with all blood types. She finds that this results in stabilizing blood sugar, improving thyroid function, a more efficient immune system and even weight loss.

Marie affirms that Coconut Oil should replace all other oils in the diet as the beneficial results are so multifaceted.

Other Uses for Coconut Oil:
Skin Care...

Used by Polynesian women for thousands of years, raw Coconut Oil has a small molecular structure, which allows it to be easily absorbed by the skin and its underlying structure, giving it a soft, smooth texture. An excellent exfoliant, Coconut Oil also aids in the removal of dead skin cells from the top layer of skin, while strengthening the underlying tissue. Leave on face for 15 minutes then wash off with Castille or Neutrogena soap.

Eye and Face Makeup Remover...

Coconut Oil is the best eyeliner and mascara remover I have ever used. I put some on my index finger and rub lightly across my eyes for a few minutes. Then, using a warm wet tissue, I just wipe away the dissolved makeup.

I also spread some Coconut Oil over my face each night to remove my foundation. It slightly exfoliates but more importantly it deeply nourishes the skin with good fat. After 5 minutes, I wipe off the excess with a warm washcloth or use an olive oil soap. It leaves my skin clean, soft and smooth.

Beauty Mask...

61

Twice a week, I make a mask of raw Coconut Oil, raw honey, 7 drops of fresh lemon juice and the contents of one vitamin E gel capsule. I spread it all over my face and neck and let it sit for about 60 minutes. Rinse off with warm water. Glowing skin will be your thank you.

RESOURCES:

The brand of Coconut Oil I used was *Tropical Traditions Virgin Gold Label Coconut Oil* which I religiously kept right near the stove. Tropical Traditions Gold label had the highest ORAC (Oxygen Radical Absorbance Capacity) rating of all Coconut Oils I researched. Tropical Traditions coconuts are harvested in the Philippines. This company advises that it stores the coconut milk in wooden kegs, and after a few days, they manually harvest the oil which floats to the top. No chemical extraction or machines are used. It is raw, unrefined and tastes fabulous. The website for this Coconut Oil is Healthytraditions.com

As a second choice, I like *"California Gold Nutrition's Extra Virgin Coconut Oil"* from Amazon ($21 for 54 oz). Lastly, there is *Kirkland* brand *unrefined Coconut Oil* from Costco, which is the least expensive ($16 for 84 oz). They all taste like butter when melted, especially the first 2 brands. They also have a shelf life of years.

- *I warn you NOT to buy any old no-name-brand Coconut Oil off a grocery store shelf, as it may have a much different taste and inferior quality than the ones I am attesting to here. I once bought one from a grocery store that smelled and tasted like rancid blue cheese. It was awful. I'm quite sure it couldn't cure a thing. Please, spare yourself the disappointment.*

Summing Up the Wisdom…

Coconut Oil is a staple in the diet of most Polynesian, Melanesian and many African and Asian diets. For hundreds of years, it has been used worldwide not only as a health food, but as a healing medicine and disease preventative. These cultures consistently exhibit far better overall health and longevity than the low-fat, bad fat-eating population of the western world. *Many of these cultures consumed up to 50% daily fat from Coconut Oil. Yet decades of documentation confirm that these civilizations have thrived in robust health and vitality for generations, virtually free from all the degenerative diseases of the western populations.* Since the 1920's, Scientific evidence has unanimously concluded that:

- *Cultures whose diets were very high in good saturated fat from raw Coconut Oil were lean and strong, living long lives of exceptional health, free from Western diseases.*

These facts have been confirmed and recorded by the following Researchers and Experts in their field:

Jon J. Kabara, Ph.D. Professor Emeritus of Chemistry and Pharmacology, Michigan State University; Dr. Weston A. Price, Founder of the Weston A. Price Foundation for Health; Dr. Ian Prior, Harvard University; Dr Julian Whitaker of the Whitaker Wellness Center and a multitude of other Health Institutions *have confirmed that those civilizations which eat Coconut Oil as their daily staple "are virtually free of all degenerative diseases."*

In a deluge of documentation over a 90 year period by multitude of Scientists and Ph.D.'s who are experts in the field of Lipids (Fats), the scientific consensus is as follows:

- *There is a critical difference between "good saturated fat" and "bad saturated fat."*

- *Coconut Oil is a Good Saturated Fat. It is life-giving, healing and strengthening to the thyroid and immune system, while also providing a biological defense against a multitude of pathogens and diseases.*

  Conversely, processed oils and hydrogenated oils have the complete opposite effect on your body, causing obesity, ill health and disease.

- **It's not about <u>reducing</u> the fat in your diet.**
  It's about <u>replacing</u> the fat in your diet.

Bad Fat...

- *Processed oils and hydrogenated oils promote and sustain ill health.*
  Processed oils and hydrogenated oils weaken the immune system, suppress thyroid function, disable insulin receptors on the cell wall so that nutrients (glucose) cannot enter the cell. That cell wall hardens and cannot receive food or eject waste. The cell eventually sickens and dies. This results in diabetes, neuropathy, hardening of the arteries and cardiovascular disease.

- Specifically, Soybean oil contains *Goitrogens, an anti-thyroid chemical* shown to suppress thyroid function, decreases metabolism and induces weight gain.

- *Processed polyunsaturated oils produced the most and the largest cancerous tumors in monkeys given cancer-causing chemicals.*
  (Cohen & Thompson, 1987; Reddy, 1992)

Good Fat…

- *Unrefined Coconut Oil strengthens the immune system, improves thyroid function, brain and eye health and optimizes the function of every cell in the body. It has the unique ability to penetrate the wall of even sick and diseased cells. By entering these cells and delivering food and nutrients, the sick or starving cell is then fed and resuscitated.*

- *Extensive studies show when cancer is chemically induced in lab animals, the type of fat in their diet determines the resulting number and size of the tumors which developed. Coconut Oil was shown to block cancer and tumor development in monkeys given cancer-causing chemicals.*
  (Cohen & Thompson, 1987; Reddy, 1992.)

- *Lauric Acid is the strongest antimicrobial Fatty Acid found in Nature. Coconut Oil has the highest Lauric Acid content of any food.*

- *Unlike processed oils, Coconut Oil does NOT store as fat. It is taken up by the liver and converted into energy and Ketones, a superfuel for brain cells.*

- *Coconut Oil kills many pathogens in the body without causing any damage to healthy cells. It is all natural and has the added benefit of having no negative side effects or interaction with medications.*

Short Version:
- *Processed and hydrogenated vegetable oils promote cell malfunction, cell death, sickness, disease and weight gain.*
- *Unrefined Coconut Oil feeds and resuscitates sick cells, combats infection and prevents disease while promoting weight loss.*

Despite 9 decades of documentation on the remarkable rewards of Coconut Oil, there are very few doctors today who will hail its benefits. Instead, they will probably warn you that it is a saturated fat and is therefore automatically bad for you and for your heart. *They erroneously believe that all saturated fats are the same. But please remember, a multitude of lipid experts from around the world have confirmed this assumption is the absolute opposite of the truth. There are thousands of studies, experiments and research findings which document that virgin Coconut Oil is a powerful healer and disease preventative, which actually supports the heart and cardiovascular system. These same lipid experts confirm it is in fact processed and hydrogenated vegetable oils (including margarine) that are in fact the major contributors to obesity, heart disease, stroke, diabetes and arteriosclerosis.*

- *Mary Enig, Ph.D. Lipid Specialist confirms the MCFA's in Coconut Oil heal the body at the cellular level and also fights against infections and disease.*

66

- *Dr. Mary Newport attests that her husband's cholesterol and blood pressure actually dropped when she put him on Coconut Oil. His Alzheimer's symptoms were reversed… and he lost 10 pounds.*

- *Dr. Bruce Fife, C.N., N.D. affirms that Coconut Oil is unlike any other fat, insofar as it protects against heart disease, cancer, diabetes and a host of other degenerative illnesses, strengthens the immune system and battles against any microbes that invade the body. It also has the distinctive capability of inducing weight loss. Dr. Fife concluded, "I found out that Coconut Oil was one of the most remarkable health foods available."*
  (Fife, 2013)

NEXT ACTION:
"Follow the Recipe,"
…1,2,3…

1 > Plug the Holes in Your Boat…
- ***ELIMINATE ALL PROCESSED OILS AND FATS FROM YOUR KITCHEN:***
  Margarine (100% hydrogenated soybean oil)
  Salad dressings that have soybean or canola oil
  Packaged snacks that have processed or hydrogenated oils in them
  Choose instead:
  Snacks like baked chips, crackers, pretzels

or oil free salad dressings, which can be purchased at health food stores like Martindale's, Sprouts, Mothers or Whole Foods.

2 > MAKE AN "OIL CHANGE"...

- **REPLACE ALL PROCESSED OILS WITH UNREFINED COCONUT OIL.**

EAT 5-8 Tablespoons of unrefined Coconut Oil a day by using it like butter, on your potatoes, on hot veggies, in your oatmeal, on your toast, in hot tea, in hot chocolate, in protein smoothies. Cook with it.

Replace unhealthy soybean oil salad dressings with oil free dressings.

FYI: Coconut Oil becomes solid at temperatures below 76 degrees, so it is not usually used in salad dressings, which are often kept refrigerated.

3 > READ THE LABEL ...

- **CHOOSE NOT TO BUY FOODS WITH PROCESSED OILS IN THEM.**
  Especially Soybean and hydrogenated oils.

You are the *Gatekeeper* of your family's health. So please make it a habit to *read the label* of all bottled, boxed and canned foods before you buy them. Ingredients are *listed in order of predominant weight or quantity*, meaning the main ingredients are the first 3-5 that are listed. Each additional ingredient is less and less in amount, the further down the list you read. *So if the first 5 ingredients have soybean oil, canola oil, palm oil or hydrogenated anything in it...put it back on the shelf.*

Simply look for a healthier alternative for that item. Almost every grocery store has a health food aisle to find alternative healthier snacks. By simply making it a habit to read the label of packaged food products, you will be controlling the direction of your family's health.

Think about it…

How many times a day do you put food or drink into your body? If almost everything you eat has unhealthy ingredients, it does not take long before the body's defenses weaken and it starts to break down, succumbing to sickness and disease.

What would happen if you put the wrong kind of gas into your car?

The engine starts to sputter and stall and simply can not function properly. Well, at least if you ruin the engine of your car, you can buy a new one; but not with your body. We get only one per customer. By simply *reading the label*, you are *taking control of your health by making an informed and conscious decision before you buy* food products containing ingredients which will break down your body's engine.

So *yes, you can take the wheel here, by choosing to put "healthy fuel" into your body to shift it into optimal performance.*

The Bible states, *"My people perish for lack of knowledge."* Now that you have finished the first chapter of this book, you are in possession of a *great deal of knowledge.* I encourage you to put it to its best use.

Change your health and your life by simply the Following the Recipe above. By choosing 3 very simple actions, you are enabling and empowering yourself to make a profound difference in your health…and in your life.

The Key to Your Best Health
…is You.

Chapter Two

"THE BLOOD OF THE PLANT"
Essential Oils

What are Essential Oils …?

Known as the "Blood of the Plant", Essential Oils are the life-giving liquid extracted from plant leaves, roots, flowers and seeds. It is undisputed that for centuries, Essential Oils from plants have been used by ancient cultures to elevate the mind and heal the body.

Essential Oils are the most concentrated and most powerful part of the plant. They are chemically complex, comprised of hundreds of bioactive compounds which collectively effect their powerful therapeutic healing. Because these oils are highly concentrated, they are far more potent than dried herbs. In some cases, you may get only a single drop of Essential Oil from an entire plant. They are very high in life-giving oxygen. Although they are called "oils", many of them are very water-like in consistency and are not at all greasy. Unlike vegetable oils, Essential Oils have a unique way of passing easily through the skin. Their consistency and chemical composition are so compatible with our blood that *our bodies literally drink them in* when they are applied topically. In this simple manner, they have the ability to instantly deliver oxygen into our cells. *Oxygenating the cells expedites healing.*

When applied to the skin, Essential Oil molecules are absorbed rapidly into the body. Some oils increase lymph and blood flow reducing inflammation, while others provide pain relief and promote tissue regeneration. In some cases, they detoxify the body or prevent infection from invading microbes and fungi. The ability of Essential Oils to quickly impact the brain, the mood and the body makes them truly unique among all other natural therapeutic agents.

History of Essential Oils...

Essential Oils are one of the oldest healing modalities in existence. Records dating back to 4,500 B.C. describe the use of Essential Oils for religious and rituals and medical application. The Egyptians were masters in using Essential Oils in both their spiritual and embalming rituals. Imhotep, the Grand Vizier to King Zeser (2780-2720 BC), is often given the credit for furthering the use of Essential Oils for medicinal purposes. Hieroglyphics found on the walls of Egyptian temples depict the blending of Essential Oils, including hundreds of recipes for healing. In the Temple of Edfu was found an ancient papyrus on which was recorded Essential Oil medicinal formulas and perfume recipes used by the alchemists and high priests for healing of the body, for emotional cleansing and for elevating the spirit.

The Egyptians used Essential oils, resins and spices in everyday life. Oils and pastes from plants were transformed into pills, powders and suppositories, medicine cakes and ointments for healing. Special blends were made for meditation, love and war. Essential oil gums were used in their embalming process and traces of them have been found on mummies today.

The Egyptians were the first to discover the potent effects of fragrance. They created various aromatic blends to be used for personal use, emotional empowerment and for the ceremonies performed in their temples. Ancient manuscripts and drawings also document the use of Essential Oils by Cleopatra in her bath, as a massage oil and as perfume. Well before the time of Christ, Egyptians collected Essential Oils and put them in alabaster vessels. These vessels were specially carved and shaped for storing the Essential Oils. In 1922, when King Tut's tomb was discovered, 350 liters of Essential oils were found there, stored inside alabaster jars. Each jar was sealed with wax, perfectly preserving the 3,200-year-old oils.

Around 3,000 B.C., a system of natural healing called Ayurvedic Medicine was developed by Indian scholars. Ayurvedic Medicine is a well-known Empirical source of Holistic Healing Modalities, still widely used today. This Ancient and revered Healing System includes Essential Oils in its treatments. Vedic literature incorporates Essential Oils into their medicinal potions, listing over 700 treatments that include cinnamon, ginger, myrrh, and sandalwood as effective for healing.

In China, the use of Essential Oils was first recorded between 2697-2597 B.C. during the reign of Emperor Huang Ti, known as the "Yellow Emperor." His famous book, *The Yellow Emperor's Book of Internal Medicine*, contains healing applications for Essential Oils, still considered useful by Eastern medicine today.

The Greek physician Hippocrates (460-377 B.C.) known as the *"Father of Medicine*," recorded the effects of approximately 300 plants and Essential Oils, including Thyme, Saffron, Marjoram, Cumin and Peppermint.

73

Hippocrates extensive knowledge of plants and Essential Oils derived from Greek soldiers' encounters with Ayurvedic medicine during their travels with Alexander the Great. Hippocrates wrote, *"A perfumed bath and scented oil massage every day is the way to good health."* His literature contains the most important principle in modern medicine:

- *"Above all, the purpose of a doctor is to awaken the natural healing energies within the body."*

Galen was another Greek Scholar who reportedly had a vast knowledge of plant Essential Oil healing. He began as a surgeon to the Gladiators. It was reputed that no gladiator died of infected wounds while Galen was surgeon. He was then promoted to personal physician to Roman Emperor Marcus Aurelius. He documented a great deal of his successful work with Essential Oils and plants in healing and averting infection. He divided plants into various medicine categories that are still known as the *"Galenic"* system today.

The Romans were well known for applying Essential Oils to their bodies, bath, bedding and clothes. They even made special blends to empower them for battle. Roman physicians took books from Galen and Hippocrates when they fled during the fall of the Roman Empire and these texts were later translated into Persian, Arabic and other languages.

The Bible records many instances where Essential Oils were used for religious ceremonies, spiritual upliftment, purification and healing, including uses of Myrrh, Frankincense, Cassia, Cinnamon and Sandalwood.

In Persia, a child Prodigy named Ali-ibn Sana (Avicenna the Arab) lived from 980 to 1037 A.D. He became a well-educated physician by the age of 12. He wrote books on the healing properties of 800 plants and Essential Oils, and documented other positive effects they had on the body. He is credited as being the first person to discover and record the unique method of distilling Essential Oils. These methods are still in use today.

In Europe during the Crusades, the Knights were responsible for passing on knowledge of Essential Oil and herbal medicine they learned in the Middle East. The Knights acquired knowledge of distillation and carried Essential Oils with them.

During the outbreak of the Bubonic Plague, Ayurvedic recipes were successfully used to ward off infection. Essential Oils of Frankincense and Pine were burned in the streets during the Plague. It was recorded that substantially less people died in the areas where this was done.

"Tell Us About the Thieves…!"

In the fifteenth century during the Bubonic Plague, it was discovered that a band of perfumers was wandering around stealing valuables from the many dead and dying bodies, yet they did not contract the deadly plague themselves. These perfumers were captured and interrogated to learn how they were impervious to the Plague. They divulged that they made a potion of Essential Oils which they rubbed on their face and clothes and even put in their mouths to successfully avert infection. This potion was a powerful blend of Essential Oils of Clove, Cinnamon, Lemon, Eucalyptus and Rosemary. This exact blend is made and sold today by Young Living Essential Oils, and it is appropriately called *"Thieves."*

This therapeutic blend was tested by Weber State University for its potent antimicrobial properties. *The study confirmed this potent blend of Essential Oils was highly antiviral, antibacterial, antiseptic and anti-infectious. The*

Thieves' blend was also found to have a 99.96% kill rate against airborne bacteria.

Stunning Discovery…

In 1928, a French Chemist named Rene-Maurice Gattefosse accidentally discovered the powerful healing properties of Essential Oils when a small explosion happened in his laboratory. He records that his hands were literally in flames. After extinguishing the flames, he was horrified to see that both his hands were covered in "rapidly developing gas gangrene." In short, the flesh on his hands began to die. He quickly ran to immerse his burnt hands into the nearest container of liquid. Turns out that liquid was Essential Oil of Lavender. *To his astonishment he found that the pain quickly dissipated from his hand. Healing began the very next day. He also had no subsequent infection and no residual scarring from his severe burn.*

Gattefosse conducted further studies on the healing properties of Lavender Oil confirming it was analgesic, antiseptic, antiviral and bactericidal and hypotensive (lowers stress and blood pressure). He then introduced this knowledge to many hospitals in France. During the outbreak of Spanish Flu, there were no reported deaths of personnel in those hospitals where Lavender Essential Oil was widely used.

Gattefosse first coined the term *"Aromatherapie"* while researching the antiseptic properties of Essential Oils. His book *Aromatherapie* details many successful results of Essential Oil healings. This book greatly influenced the healing practices in France.

During World War II, a Parisian doctor named Jean Valnet recorded that he resorted to using Essential Oils to treat the wounded soldiers when he had run out of antibiotics. To his great surprise, he found that the Essentials Oils were able to reduce and even stop infection.

"How do I use Essential Oils...?"
There are 5 very simple ways of using Essential Oils:

1. Ingestion:
The French preferred ingestion of Essential Oils by way of putting a drop on a sugar cube or by putting a drop of lemon oil or peppermint oil in drinks.
- **Please Note: Not all Essential Oils are SAFE TO EAT.**

Before ingesting an Essential oil, you must first ascertain that it has a "GRAS" designation from FDA which means it is "Generally Regarded as Safe to Eat." (Young Living Essential Oils have many Oils with a GRAS designation.)

2. Inhalation:
The Germans recommended inhalation of Essential Oils. This is achieved by using a diffuser which atomizes the oil, shooting droplets into the air. Putting Lavender and Lemon Essential Oils in a diffuser on your nightstand is an excellent way to mitigate snoring, induce deeper sleep and also disinfects the air of your bedroom.

You can also put a few drops of Peppermint Oil in the palm of your hands, briefly touch your palms together, and cup your hands over your nose and mouth. Then breath in deeply through your nose and out your mouth 10x. This will effectively open up stuffy nasal passages and disinfect sinuses.

3. Bath:

Adding Essential Oils to your bath delivers benefits to your body in two ways:
The steam causes the oil molecules to enter your nose as you breathe, then passing quickly through your olfactory bulb and into various parts of the brain. Also, your skin readily absorbs the Essential Oil from the bath water.

4. Direct Topical Application:

Direct topical application is also very effective. Later in this chapter I will go into more detail about how to directly apply *1-2 drops of specific Essential Oils* to cuts, sprains, burns, gum infections or to the back and chest to relieve congestion, coughing and to reduce fever.

5. Massage:

Essential Oils can be *added to a carrier oil,* like pure Coconut Oil, Olive oil or Almond Oil to be used to massage the body for relaxation, muscle pain relief or stress relief.

How Essential Oils Heal...

Essential Oils heal in two ways: *They are high in Oxygen and Frequency.*

Oxygen:
The Giver of Life...

You may remember from grade school science class the term *"Photosynthesis"* which is the process by which plants use sunlight, carbon dioxide and water *to generate oxygen.* This is why plant Essential Oils are so high in oxygen. Due to their many bioactive components, Essential Oils are remarkably compatible with our blood. As mentioned previously, when applied to our skin, our bodies literally drink them in. Essential Oils are made up of tiny molecules which easily penetrate the skin and other body systems, very quickly making their way into the bloodstream. Many Essential Oils contain compounds that fight harmful bacteria, viruses and fungi, while others contain components that ease pain, reduce inflammation and heal wounds.

All Essential Oils deliver oxygen directly into the cells of the applied area. Oxygen is an all-natural healer. Essential Oils are unique in that you can apply them to a specific target area or wound to effect healing through the immediate oxygenation of those injured or sick cells.

Biology of the Brain…

When inhaled, Essential Oils have the unique ability to pass through the nose and through the Olfactory Bulb which connects to the brain's Hypothalamus, Thalamus, Pituitary Gland, Pineal Gland, Amygdala and Hippocampus. In short, it passes easily into the *Command Center* of the brain.

The Hypothalamus is the hormone command center of the body as well as the control center for thirst, hunger and mood. The Limbic System of the brain, known as the *seat of emotions,* includes the Amygdala and the Hippocampus. This area is responsible for behavioral and emotional responses. Collectively, these areas of the brain *are directly affected by inhaling Essential Oils.* How these areas are affected depends upon which oils you are inhaling. Some Essential Oils, like Lemon and Lavender, will have a greatly relaxing and calming effect, while oils like Peppermint and Cinnamon will increase focus and alertness.

Other Essential Oils, like Frankincense and Myrrh have been shown to *dramatically increase oxygenation and activity of the brain when inhaled.* These remarkable Oils have a component called *Sesquiterpenes* which amazingly enables them to pass easily *through the blood-brain barrier.* This powerful and unique capability may help you understand why decades of research has confirmed that inhaling Essential Oils *exerts a powerful effect on the brain*, including the ability to balance mood and emotions. The regular use of Essential Oils to achieve and maintain physical and mental health is a simple *Holistic Healing Practice* that is unique, powerful and direct.

"What is Frequency...?"
Surprise...our Bodies are Electrical.

Frequency is the measurable rate of electrical energy flow. It is the measurement of one wave cycle of electricity measured in Hertz (Hz), which equals one wave cycle per second. Every cell in our body is specialized to conduct electrical current. This electrical current is needed for the nervous system to send signals throughout the brain and body, making it possible for us to move, think and feel. Hence, it is crucial for athletes to drink *electrolytes* to avoid depletion after strenuous exertion of energy. A steady heartbeat depends on balanced electrolytes as do hundreds of other functions of the body, right down to our cellular activity.

The brain uses chemicals and electrical impulses to communicate. These electrical impulses can travel up to 120 meters per second. A neuron is a nerve cell that transmits and receives signals from your brain, muscles and glands. *We have over 100 billion neurons in our brain which send and receive signals.* These neurons use *electrical signals to communicate* with each other and with the body. This is referred to as an *Electrochemical Charge.* This charge changes according to need, depending on whether the neuron is resting or sending a signal.

Everything we do is controlled and enabled by electrical signals running through our bodies. You couldn't read this book without them. Your brain sends a neural electrochemical impulse at warp speed to tell your hand to swat away a fly that just landed on your face. Many electrical signals are almost instantaneous, saving us from life and death situations like jumping out of the way of a car. You don't "think" about jumping out of the way. Your brain simply sends a neural impulse (*electrochemical* signal) to the neurons in your leg muscles (motor neurons) causing them to contract and instantaneously jump according to the signal. If someone is chasing you, the brain instantly and automatically sends an electrical impulse signal releasing cortisol, the *"flight or fight"* hormone. This instantly increases your heart rate and muscle strength to adapt to the perceived threat. All in all, the body is the most amazing and fascinating machine. All we have to do is to take good care of it, and it will serve us long and well.

In our home, electricity flows through wires; but in our body it rapidly flows through chains of cells until it reaches its destination. When the initial electrical impulse is sent, it *"fires"* through the necessary cell path, reaching its destination by way of a *chain reaction*. We all learned in Physics that everything is made of up atoms, which are either positively charged, negatively charged or neutral. *Our bodies are composed of trillions of these charged atoms which enable us to generate electricity*. Our cells exchange information and regulate body functions through the sending and receiving of information via specific frequencies levels of electricity.

- Maintaining high Frequency ensures the body successfully sends and receives the critical signals which regulate all life-sustaining actions.

Studies performed at Johns Hopkins University confirmed that the *lower the frequency of the body, the greater the risk of disease.* It was further discovered that the use of pure therapeutic grade *Essential Oils substantially raises both the Frequency and Oxygen levels of the body,* making it difficult if not impossible for most microbes to multiply.

Think about mosquitoes. Wetlands and marshy areas with tall grass *invite them* to breed there. *Why?* Because the *environment is favorable for their reproduction.* Conversely, *we can choose to easily create "an unfavorable environment" for microbe breeding by keeping our Oxygen and Frequency levels high.*

Gimme the Short Version…

- *When your body's frequency is low, the cells cannot "communicate" at their optimal capacity. This causes biochemical actions to slow down or break down at the cellular level. In turn, the body's cells and organs break down and eventually deteriorate.*

- *Low body Frequency invites and allows microbes to multiply.*

- *Microbes cannot multiply in a High-Frequency, High-Oxygen environment.*

- Therapeutic grade *Essential Oils substantially raise both the Frequency and Oxygen levels of the body.*

- *Keeping the body at its highest Frequency is a very powerful way to keep it functioning at its highest efficiency while also keeping sickness at bay.*

The Science:
Using Frequency to Heal and Prevent Disease...

In the early 1920s, a "Frequency Generator" was developed by Dr Royal Raymond Rife. He found that by using *certain frequencies (levels of electrical energy) he was able to kill a virus or cancer cell.* He further discovered that these same frequencies *could prevent* the development of disease, while other frequencies would *destroy disease.*

Dr. Royal Rife documented the following:

"*For many years during my clinical practice, I researched the use of electrical energy for the purpose of reversing the disease process. I kept feeling there must be a more natural way of increasing a person's electrical frequency, which led to my discovery of the electrical frequency of essential oils.*

One of the things I noticed with my patients was that they felt better emotionally when they first started to use essential oils. Also, it seemed that within seconds, congestion would begin to loosen just through the simple inhalation of an oil. Certain oils applied on location would decrease pain 50-80% within 1-3 minutes. Some patients even experienced a decrease in pain within seconds. I could not have thought that an oil applied to the bottom of the feet could travel to the neck and reduce pain by 70% within 1 minute. As I saw this happen over and over, I started to realize that there had to be aspects and elements in Essential Oils that had to be researched." (Rife, 2018)

Dr. Rife believed that:

- *"Every disease has a frequency, and a substance with a Higher Frequency will alter the disease which is at a lower frequency." (Rife, 2018)*

Scientists in the field of natural healing agreed there must be a natural way to increase the body's frequency/electrical energy defense against disease. This belief triggered the research and subsequent discovery of the electrical Frequency of pure Essential Oils.

In 1992, Bruce Tainio of Tainio Technology, a division of Washington Eastern State University, built the world's first Frequency monitor. With this device, Tainio determined that the average frequency of a healthy human body was between 62-78 Hertz (Hz).

- *He further confirmed that when body frequency drops, the immune system becomes compromised.*

If body frequency drops to 60 Hz, colds and flu symptoms appear. Frequency below 58 Hz exposes the body to disease. His findings were as follows:

Brain frequency of a genius:	80-82 Hz
Normal brain frequency:	72 Hz
Healthy Human body frequency:	62-78 Hz
Thyroid and parathyroid glands:	62-68 Hz
Heart rate:	67-70 Hz
Lung frequency:	8-65 Hz
Liver frequency:	55-60 Hz

Diseases begins:	58	Hz
Candida supergrowth begins:	55	Hz
Receptivity to Epstein Barr virus:	52	Hz
Receptivity to Cancer begins:	42	Hz
Death begins:	25	Hz

Tainio also documented that everything has a frequency:

Canned foods:	0	Hz
Fresh produce, up to:	15	Hz
Dry herbs:	12-22	Hz
Fresh herbs:	20-27	Hz

Essential Oils start at 52 Hz and go as high as 420 Hz (Blue Spruce Oil).

- *Science confirms that pure Essential Oils have the highest Frequency of any natural substance known to man.*

- *The natural chemistry, Oxygen and Frequency of pure Essential Oils create an environment in which most microbes cannot live or breed.*

- *When topically applied to the feet, Pure Essential Oils can travel throughout the body in a matter of minutes.*

Our Electric Brains...

As we learned, your brain cells communicate with each other and with the body by way of electrical signals. These signals produce *electrical patterns* known as *brain waves*. An Electroencephalogram (EEG) is a test performed on the brain; whereby small electronic pads are placed on the head to measure brain wave activity. This activity is reflected on a viewing screen in real time. These brain waves have Frequencies that are measured in Hertz (Hz). This invaluable tool greatly helped scientists and doctors understand the difference between usual brain wave activity and unusual brain wave activity. The FDA approved the use of EEG tests to diagnose ADHD, attention deficit hyperactivity disorder.

Types of Brain Waves:
>*Alpha waves* reflect the brain in a relaxed state (8-12 Hz).
>
>*Beta waves* reflect the brain in normal conscious, waking states (15-22 Hz).
>
>*High Beta* waves reflect excitement or anxiousness (22-38 Hz).
>
>*Theta waves* reflect daydreaming, lost in thought, drowsy (4-8 Hz).
>
>*Delta waves* reflect a deep restorative phase of sleep (1-4 Hz).
>
>*Gamma waves* reflect a high level of thought, concentration, focus,learning and memory (30-80 Hz)

A brain that produces low frequency Gamma waves reflects lack of attention, inability to focus and possibly learning disabilities.

EEG testing has confirmed that *raising the Frequency of Gamma brain waves* causes a higher state of awareness, increases attention span, increases learning, increases memory and improves brain function overall. EEG testing further confirms that people with ADHD have some unbalanced brain waves. In short, *their Theta/Beta wave ratio is off.* We can now understand that *brain wave imbalance is a Frequency problem.* Essential Oils are the only method I know that can quickly and effectively raise and rebalance brain waves.

Seeing is Believing:
Inhaling Essential Oils Balance Brain Waves...

Many years ago, I watched an educational video showing Dr. Gary Young of Young Living Essential Oils conducting an EEG test on an ADHD child. As expected, the brain wave graph on the viewing screen reflected a continuous, high-spiking pattern of this child's Theta waves. Dr. Young then proceeded to put several drops of *pure Lemon Essential Oil* onto a small piece of cotton and tucked it into one of the child's nostrils. *Within 10 seconds, the graph of this child's brain waves dramatically reversed! Before my eyes, the child's Theta waves literally just crashed down to normal, while simultaneously, his Beta waves shot up to reach their optimal level.* In other words, *breathing in the Essential Oil of Lemon corrected this child's brain frequency and brain wave imbalance in literally 10 seconds.* It was the most amazing and impactful proof I had ever seen regarding Essential Oils' powerful and immediate effect on the brain. And, it is not something I will ever forget.

At the end of this chapter, you will find my personal testimonials on how this same simple act of inhaling Essential Oil of Lemon has made dramatic changes in the behavior of other ADHD children and of children in general.

Certain Essential Oils when inhaled can act on the brain in as little as 1 minute. When Essential Oils were diffused in hospital rooms, patients became calmer and less anxious within minutes. It is also fascinating to note that when applied to the bottom of the feet, most Essential Oils will travel throughout the body in as little as 3 minutes. *(Essential Oils Desk Reference,* 2000)

Every day of my life, I apply Essential Oils to the bottom of my feet, throat glands and spine. This is my morning habit and takes just a minute to do. At night, I diffuse Essential Oils in my bedroom while I sleep. As I sit here writing this book, I have beside me a diffuser containing pure Peppermint Oil streaming the invigorating scent of Peppermint into the air, which I am breathing in to keep my mind alert and focused. Of all the healing modalities presented in this book, I have found that the proper use of pure, therapeutic grade Essential Oils has by far the most immediate effects. Even so, I use all the Holistic Practices presented in this book for disease prevention and to maintain exceptional vigor and health. Because I believe that *our Health is our highest measure of Wealth.*

"Aren't All Essential Oils the Same...?"
That's a NO heck NO...

As with the Coconut Oil precaution in the previous chapter, I caution you against the purchase and use of just any no-name-brand, don't-know-where-it-came-from alleged Essential Oil you may find in a random health food store. Take note that many Essential Oils are sold simply to refresh the air with a pleasant scent. Beware of companies that sell what they call Essential Oils, yet they have a *"warning"* on their bottle stating: *"Not for use on the body."* Seriously...? This warning should alert you to the fact that the oil in this bottle has been altered or adulterated, possibly diluted with a chemical or some other extraneous additives causing it to be unsafe for use on the body. *This kind of oil is of no use to you at all.* If it is unsafe to apply to the body, well then I'm thinking you sure don't want to be breathing it in either.

Save your money.

The many healings I testify to at the end of this chapter resulted from the use of ONLY *100% pure Therapeutic Grade Essential Oils*, mostly *Young Living Essential Oils*. I learned that this brand properly and painstakingly distills their oils to preserve potency and rigorously tests them to confirm they are *Therapeutic Grade*. This is the purest and most powerful of any grade of Essential Oils. Also, this brand offers many types of Essential Oils that have been given the *GRAS designation*, which means they are even "safe to eat."

"Why Must I use only Therapeutic Grade Essential Oils...?"

Pure Therapeutic Grade Essential Oils are the Only Ones that Heal. Period.

Therapeutic Grade Essential Oils follow very rigid guidelines for extraction and processing. Essential Oils are derived from various parts of plants. These oils contain hundreds of naturally occurring delicate chemical compounds and elements. The measure of their purity is determined by *how well these many compounds have been preserved* throughout the extraction process and marketing process. Also*, no water or chemicals should be added* after extraction.

- *There is a world of difference between Therapeutic Grade Essential Oils and non-Therapeutic Grade Essential Oils. The first kind has potent healing properties; the second kind smells nice, but has no healing punch behind it.* Clearly, *the latter is not the caliber of Essential Oil that will change your life anytime soon.*

- *Therapeutic Grade Essential Oils are the unadulterated, purest form of Essential Oils, the most preserved and the most potent in their natural healing power.*

Proper Distillation...

Extraction of *Therapeutic Grade Essential Oils* is a diligent process which ensures purity without lessening its healing effects. Plants used should be free of any pesticides and herbicides that may adversely react with the distilled oil producing toxic compounds. The very fragile aromatic compounds within these oils are easily destroyed by high temperature and pressure or contact with certain reactive metals. This is why Therapeutic Grade Essential Oils are distilled in stainless steel cooking chambers at low temperature and low pressure. In Europe, a set of standards has been established to outline the chemical profile and principle elements that a quality Essential Oil should have. These are known as AFNOR and ISO standards. These guidelines help buyers differentiate between a Therapeutic Grade Essential Oil and an oil that is similar in fragrance and elements but is of much lower grade.

Lastly, *no scientist in any lab has been able to recreate an identical chemical profile of pure Essential Oils, which are unique in the proportions of hundreds of naturally occurring elements.*

This should help you understand why *Therapeutic Grade Essential Oils* are such a precious commodity; because their rigorous guidelines and extraction methods produce *the purest, most effective and most potent version of any Essential Oil.*

The Science of Essential Oils…

There are several similarities between Essential Oils, the *Blood of the Plant,* and human blood. They both fight infection, contain hormone-like compounds and initiate regeneration and healing. Essential Oils serve as the chemical defense mechanism of the plant, possessing potent antibacterial, antiviral and antifungal properties. Certain Essential Oils have hormone-like compounds which have the ability to bring physiological balance to many systems of the body. For example, Clary Sage and Fennel have an estrogenic action.

The unique lipid-soluble structure of Essential Oils is very similar to the make-up of our cell membranes. Essential Oil molecules are very tiny, giving them the ability to *penetrate every cell with ease.* It is fascinating to note that Essential Oils have a chemical structure very similar to that found in human blood and tissues. This unique feature allows Essential Oils to be compatible with and easily accepted by the human body, whereby the body literally drinks these oils in through the skin.

This gives Essential Oils the powerful ability to diffuse through tissue and blood. They powerfully penetrate the membrane of any sick cell, healing it with oxygen and Frequency.
…Just think about the power in that.

Researchers further discovered that diffusing Essential Oils into the air increases atmospheric oxygen and provides negative ions which inhibit the growth of bacteria.

Only about 10% are used for medicine and therapeutic applications. Approximately 90% of the Essential Oils produced today are used for the perfume industry.

Applications…

Because Essential Oils are a composite of many different chemical elements, they each have remarkable and unique effects on the mind and body. For example, Clove Oil is both antiseptic and anesthetic when applied topically. It can also be anti-tumoral. Clove oil was used for decades by Dentists to *numb the gums* and to prevent infection. Lavender Oil has been effectively used for burns, wound healing, insect bites, anxiety, insomnia, stress and to increase hair growth. Imagine having all these benefits from just one kind of Essential Oil, with no negative side effects.

Moreover, because of their compatibility with human blood, Essential Oils do not disturb the body's natural physical and chemical balance, or homeostasis. Even when applied to only one part of the body, they travel throughout the entire body in minutes, raising the body's Oxygen and Frequency. Whereas, synthetic chemicals, like prescription drugs, most often have only one action, and usually disrupts or negatively affects the body's overall health.

Actions Essential Oils Trigger in the Body…

In the human body, pure Essential Oils stimulate the secretion of antibodies, neurotransmitters, endorphins, hormones and enzymes. Oils containing *limonene* have been shown to be anti-viral. Other oils like Lavender and Roman Chamomile, have been shown to regenerate skin and very effectively heal wounds. Essential Oils increase the uptake of oxygen and ATP (adenosine triphosphate), fuel for every cell in the body. European scientists discovered some

Essential Oils have the ability to work as natural *chelators,* binding with heavy metals and carrying them out of the body.

Most Essential Oils have some combination of following benefits:

> *Analgesic* properties which ease pain
> A*ntiseptic* properties which prevent or heal infections
> A*nti-inflammatory* properties
> C*alming* and promoting sleep
> S*timulating,* promoting focus
> *Hormone secretion*
> *Reduce fever*
> *Relieve congestion*
> *Antimicrobial, kills germs*
> *All Essential Oils raise Oxygen and Frequency.*

Let me say here that by acquiring and maintaining a basic collection of these health-giving oils, you will have compiled a *powerful arsenal of prevention and healing* that will serve you and your family, for life.

Instruction for Use…

The Essential Oil bottles come with a diffusing insert so that the oil does not *spill* out of the bottle; it comes out in drops. You simply tilt the open bottle, putting *one drop* of precious oil onto your fingertip*. Apply this drop immediately to the affected area, before your fingertip drinks it in.*

These oils are very potent, therefore "*less is more.*"

Direct Application to the Skin:

To treat a cut, scrape, bruise, insect bite, mole, wart or local skin infection simply put 1-2 drops of Essential Oil

93

onto your index fingertip and then *dab or briefly spread* the oil onto the target area. *DO NOT RUB IT IN*, as your skin on your fingers will drink in the oil in seconds. Using more than 1-2 drops on a small area will be just wasting the oil.

Fresh Burn:

Apply 1 drop of *Lavender Oil* to burn, wait 5 minutes and repeat. Wait another 5 minutes and apply a third drop. This triple application within 15 minutes is used to reduce pain when the burn is fresh and very painful. Thereafter, apply one drop 3x a day till healed. Do not put any cream or other chemical on top of the Lavender Oil.

Insect Bites:

Apply 1 drop Lavender Oil or *Purification* (YLEO blend) 3x a day.

Warts or Moles:

Apply 1 drop of *Frankincense* + 1 drop of *Lemon Oil* 3-4x a day.

Cut, Scrape, Bruise:

Apply 1 drop *Lavender Oil* 2-3x a day.

Large area Bruise:

Mix 2 drops of *Lavender Oil or 2 drops Lemongrass Oil with 1 Tbsp Coconut Oil* and spread over the area.

Muscle Ache:

2 drops *Birch Oil, Wintergreen or Lavender Oil* 2x a day

Pulled Ligament:

2 drops of *Lemongrass Oil* 3x a day

Skin Rash:

4 drops *Lavender Oil* mixed with 1 Tbsp *Coconut Oil*; mix and spread over the rash. (It's important to identify the source of the rash. Because, if it's a food allergy, it will soon return.)

Pilonidal Cyst / Cyst / Abscess:

1 drop of *Frankincense Oil* + 1 drop of *Lemon Oil* 4x a day

Gum Abscess:

1 drop *Clove Oil*

- *This is a very strong oil! Can be diluted with Coconut Oil.*

Fever Blisters:

1 drop *Melaleuca Oil* 3x a day

Boils: 1 drop *Roman Chamomile Oil* 3-4x a day

Toenail fungus:

1 drop *Melaleuca Oil* + 1 drop *Eucalyptus Oil* 3x a day

Athlete's foot:

Mix 2 drops each of *Melaleuca Oil and Eucalyptus Oil with* 2 Tbsp *Coconut Oil* and massage onto your feet.

- Put socks on before walking as feet may be slightly slippery.
- *Athlete's foot is a fungal infection. I strongly suggest that you eat 4-8 Tbsp per day of raw Coconut Oil to rid the entire body of the fungal cause.*

Acne:

1 drop *Eucalyptus Oil* + 1 drop *Lavender Oil* mixed with 3 tablespoons pure Aloe Vera Gel. Spread on the affected area 2x a day.

- After applying to face, close your eyes and fan your face with any small cardboard or piece of paper, as these oils will make your eyes water for a few minutes. Fan your face til the scent dissipates. It's well worth it.

- *Please Note:* Acne is caused by the *acnes bacteria* living in the body. These bacteria will have to be eradicated systemically for permanent relief. I strongly suggest *eating 5-8 Tbsp a day of raw Coconut Oil* a day. You can put it on any food, on toast, in tea or in a smoothie to help *rid the body of these bacteria.* Otherwise, breakouts may recur.

Headache:

1 drop of *Frankincense* on each temple or 2 drops *Peppermint Oil* on back of neck

Acid Reflux:

1 drop *Peppermint Oil* in a 10 oz glass of water.

Drink with straw because oil floats.

Acid Indigestion:
Put 1 drop of *Peppermint Oil* in 10 oz water. Drink with straw as oil floats.

> Contrary to popular belief, <u>chronic indigestion is often due to LOW stomach acid.</u> Therefore, the *Peppermint Oil* will solve the problem for the moment, but *you would need to correct the source of the disorder for it to go away permanently.* I have helped many people accomplish this by recommending a simple over the counter natural enzyme and stomach acid support supplement called *"Super Enzymes"* by *Now* brand. This supplement contains Bromelain from pineapples and papain from papayas, as well as amylase, lipase and protease pancreas support.
> This supplement has had great success in eliminating the need for acid-reducing drugs.
> - *This supplement must be eaten WITH meals.*

What Does Each Essential Oils Do...?
There are hundreds of Essential Oils on the market today from various sellers. In the interest of time and sanity, I now give you a synopsis of 20 of my favorites which I have found to be both powerful and versatile. This will give you a great selection from which to choose when building your *"Essential Oil Arsenal"* for the healing and protection of your family. The following healing actions attributed to each specific Essential Oil are extracted from the *Essential Oil*

Desk Reference Book (2002), Essential Science Publishing, which is a compilation of detailed extensive research results regarding the remarkable effects that each of the following Essential Oils has on the body:

Essential Oil of Basil (Ocimum basilicum)
Action:
Antispasmodic (relieves muscle spasms), relaxes muscles, anti-inflammatory, anti-infectious, anti-viral, antibacterial, decongestant of veins and arteries of the lungs, increases circulation Fyfe L., et al. (1997).

Antimicrobial Agents.
Lachowitz K.J. (1998). *Lett Appl Microbiol.*

Uses:
Relax muscles, treat insect stings or bites, bronchitis and mental fatigue.
Basil may be inhaled to treat migraines and chest infections.

Application:
For sore muscles or spasm apply 1-2 drops directly to the target area.
For tension headaches, apply 1 drop to the tip of the nose and temples.
For mental fatigue, apply 1 drop to the crown of head, forehead, over heart and in navel.
Apply directly to insect bites or sting.
For chest congestion, apply 2 drops to the sternum for chest congestion, also inhale.

Inhalation:
May be directly inhaled or diffused to relieve mental fatigue

Ingestion:
Basil Oil from YLEO has GRAS designation advising it is safe to eat.
It can be added to food or drink.
- *Only Essential Oils with a GRAS designation should be ingested.*
  (Generally Regarded as Safe to Eat)

Essential Oil of Birch (Betula alleghaniensis)
Action:
Analgesic (pain killer), antispasmodic (relieves spasms), anti-inflammatory, liver stimulant, supports bone function.

Uses:
Arthritis, rheumatism, inflammation, muscle pain, tendonitis, cramps contains an active compound similar to cortisone and is beneficial for bone, muscle and joint discomfort.

Application:
Apply 1-2 drops directly to the target area to relieve pain. Can be mixed with carrier oil (coconut oil or almond oil) to be used on a large area of the body or as a massage oil.

Inhalation:
May be directly inhaled or diffused. Stimulates and increases awareness in all levels of sensory system.

Essential Oil of Cinnamon Bark (Cinnamomum verum)
Action:
Highly antimicrobial, anti-infectious, antibacterial for a large spectrum of infection, antiviral, antifungal (Candida), sexual

stimulant, increases blood flow Tantaoui-Elaraki A., et al. (1994). *J. Environ Pathol Toxicol Oncol.*

History:
Cinnamon Oil is one of the most powerful antimicrobial Essential Oils. It has been successfully used for over 2,000 years. Research has found that *pathogenic organisms cannot live in the presence of Cinnamon Oil* (Yousef, 1980).

Uses:
Increase circulation, combat infections, respiratory infections, digestion, exhaustion, rheumatism and to treat warts, typhoid, infectious disease, sexual stimulant

Application:
Apply 2 drops under the ball and heel of feet and to ankles
> **Caution: Cinnamon Oil is very strong!**
- DO NOT DIRECTLY APPLY TO SKIN UNDILUTED, except under ball and heel of feet (where skin is thickest)
- Can be mixed with coconut oil or almond oil to dilute
- If overapplication causes you to itch, put coconut oil, almond oil or olive oil over the affected area for relief.

Inhalation:
May be diffused for upper respiratory illness and mental stimulation.

Ingestion:
Cinnamon Oil from YLEO has GRAS designation advising it is safe to eat.
It can be added to food or drink.

- *Only Essential Oils with a GRAS designation should be ingested.*
  (Generally Regarded as Safe to Eat)

Essential Oil of Clary Sage (Salvia sclarea)
Action:
Contains Phytoestrogens (estrogen-like plant compounds) that help balance female hormones, anti-infectious, antifungal, antispasmodic (relieves spasms), antibacterial, relaxing, treats menopausal and PMS symptoms

Uses:
Hormone imbalance, insomnia, hemorrhoids, menstrual cramps, PMS, pre-menopause, menopause symptoms

Application:
Apply 1-2 drops to ankles and wrists.

Inhalation:
May be directly inhaled or diffused to promote calm and sleep.

Essential Oil of Clove (Syzygium aromaticum)
Action:
Highly antimicrobial, antiseptic, analgesic (pain killer), bactericidal (kills bacteria), anti-inflammatory, disinfectant, hemostatic (blood thinning), insecticidal.
   Nishijima H., et al. (1999). *Jpn J Pharmacol.*

History:
On the Indonesian Island of Ternate, the inhabitants were known to be seemingly impervious to epidemics. They relied heavily upon the preventative powers of the Clove tree.

Dutch conquerors came and destroyed the Clove trees which naturally flourished on the island. Subsequently, the natives fell prey to the many epidemics which followed.

Clove Oil's principle ingredient, Eugenol, is used in the Dental industry for gum infections and to numb the gums.

Courmont, et al, confirmed that a solution of only .05% Eugenol from Clove Oil was sufficient to kill Tuberculosis Bacillus (Gattefosse, 1990).

According to Dr. Jean Valnet, Clove Oil is effective for prevention of many contagious diseases and successfully treats cholera, amoebic dysentery, dental infections, diarrhea, neuritis, rheumatism, bacterial colitis, viral hepatitis and warts.

"The Eugenol in Clove Oil protects nerve cells from excitotoxic and oxidative injury."

Wie, M.B., et al. (1997). *Neuroscience Lett.*

Uses:
Infectious diseases, tuberculosis, intestinal parasites, respiratory infections, toothache, scabies, wound infection shingles

Application:
Put 1 drop on infected gum or around an infected tooth.
Apply 1-2 drops under ball and heel of feet
Caution: Clove Oil is very strong!

- *DO NOT DIRECTLY APPLY TO SKIN UNDILUTED,* except under ball and heel of feet (where skin is thickest)
- *May be diluted with Coconut Oil or almond oil before applying*

- *If itching occurs, put Coconut Oil or almond oil over on affected area; NOT water, which only spreads the oil.*

Inhalation:
May be diffused: antibacterial, mentally stimulating

Essential Oil of Cypress (Cupressus sempervirens)
Action:
Improve circulation and supports nerves and intestines, anti-infectious, antimicrobial, antibacterial, strengthens blood capillary walls, strengthens connective tissue, supports pancreas and liver function

Uses:
Arthritis, bronchitis, poor circulation, hemorrhoids, menstrual pains, pancreatic insufficiency, pulmonary infections, spasms, varicose veins, fluid retention, improves skin, lessens scars, liver support

Application:
Apply 2-3 drops to swollen or sprained areas.
For circulation, apply 2-3 drops under each armpit or behind knees.
Apply 3-4 drops along spine, spread lightly with ONE finger for a few seconds only
* Do not use your palm to spread oil; it will be absorbed into your hand.

Inhalation:
May be inhaled or diffused. Promotes feeling of strength, grounding, and supports healing from emotional trauma.

Essential Oil of Eucalyptus Citriodora

Action:

Antifungal, antiseptic, antiviral, antibacterial, expectorant, deodorant, insecticidal

Weyers, W., et al. (1989). *Pharm Unserer Zeit.*

Uses:

Asthma, athlete's foot and other fungal infections, dandruff, fever, herpes, infectious skin conditions, laryngitis, shingles, sore throat

Application:

Apply 1-2 drops directly onto the target area or to the bottom of feet to treat systemic infections Apply 3-5 drops along the spine, spread lightly and briefly with one fingertip.

　　　Do Not use your palm to spread oil; it will be absorbed into your hand.

For Athletes Foot, it may be mixed with raw Coconut Oil and massaged onto feet.

Inhalation:

May be inhaled directly by putting 2 drops into the palm of hand, briefly touch palms together then cup hands over mouth and nose; breathe in deeply through the nose, exhale through the mouth 10x to open sinuses.

May be diffused: disinfectant, emotionally uplifting

Essential Oil of Eucalyptus Globulus

Action:

Antimicrobial, antifungal (candida), antiviral, antiseptic, antibacterial, expectorant, mucolytic (breaks down mucus)

Zanker, K.S., et al. (1980). *Respiration.*

History:

For centuries, Australian Aborigines used Eucalyptus leaves to dress and heal wounds. Laboratory testing confirmed Eucalyptus Globulus contains a high percentage of *Eucalyptol*, a key ingredient in many antiseptic mouthwashes sold today. Successfully used to treat respiratory disorders. Eucalyptus trees have been planted throughout parts of North Africa to successfully block the spread of Malaria. Research has also confirmed its insect-repelling properties (Trigg, 1996).

According to research done by Dr. Jean Valnet, a solution of only a 2% solution of Eucalyptus Oil sprayed into the air will kill 70% of airborne Staph bacteria.

Uses:

Acne, allergies, bronchitis, respiratory infections and disorders, sinus congestion, sinus infection, arthritis, malaria, skin and throat infections, ulcers, wounds

Application:

Apply 1-2 drops directly to the target area.

Apply to the outside of the ear, temples, back of neck, to navel or bottom of feet.

For chest congestion: Apply 2 drops onto sternum and 3 drops onto the spine, between shoulder blades.

Inhalation:

To open sinuses, may be inhaled directly by putting 2 drops into the palm of hand, briefly touch palms together, then cup hands over mouth and nose; breathe in deeply through the nose, exhale through the mouth, 10x.

May be diffused: disinfectant, emotionally uplifting

Essential Oil of Frankincense (Boswellia carteri)

Action:

Antitumoral, Immunostimulant, antimicrobial, expectorant, antidepressant, antiseptic, carminative (induces expulsion of excess gas from stomach and intestines)

History:

Frankincense has been used for centuries in the Middle East, and is known as the *"Father of all Essentials Oils."* Its use is well recorded in the Bible for healing and ceremonious anointing of a new King. Valued more than Gold, only those of great wealth possessed it. Infants of Royal birth were anointed with Frankincense to protect them from sickness and harm.

Frankincense is very high in *Sesquiterpenes* which have the unique ability to cross the blood-brain barrier, easily delivering its powerful benefits to the brain. Specifically, Frankincense stimulates the pineal gland, the Limbic portion of the brain (the seat of emotion) as well as the Hypothalamus (control center) and the Pituitary, which is the master gland of the human body that controls the release of many hormones, including thyroid and growth hormone.

Wang, L.G., Chung, K., Hsueh Pao, Y.L., et al. (1991).

Uses:

To boost Immunity, boost white blood cells, depression, headaches, bronchitis, cysts, tumors, snake bite, herpes, inflammation, typhoid, moles, warts

Application:

Apply 1-2 drops directly to the target area.
Apply 4-5 drops along the spine, spread briefly with one fingertip.

Do not spread with palm of your hand as oil will absorb into your hand

Caution: NEVER USE FRANKINCENSE ON A BURN.

Inhalation:
May be directly inhaled or diffused: strengthens immune system, improves mental focus, uplifts emotionally

Essential Oil of Geranium (Pelargonium graveolens)
Action:
Antispasmodic, antitumoral, adrenal cortex stimulant, hemostatic (stops bleeding), anti-inflammatory, antibacterial, antifungal, astringent, revitalizes skin tissue, dilates bile ducts for liver detoxification, and improves blood flow
   Fang H.J., Hsueh Pao, Y.L., et al. (1989).

Uses:
Gout, skin conditions such as dermatitis, eczema, psoriasis, herpes shingles, tumor growths, hormone imbalances, circulatory problems, liver disorders, menstrual pain, neuralgia, pancreas imbalance, ringworm, shingles, induces regeneration of tissues and nerve health Dr. Jean Valnet recommends Geranium for liver disorders and hepatitis.

Application:
Apply 1-2 drops to target area

Inhalation:
May be diffused for emotional balance, calm nerves, relieve stress

Essential Oil of Ginger (Zingiber officinale)
Action:

Anti-nausea, digestive tonic, sexual tonic, reduces pain, expectorant

Uses:
Motion sickness, nausea, arthritis, chills, respiratory infections, digestive disorders, sinusitis, sprains

Application:
May be directly applied to the target area.
For motion sickness or nausea: Apply 1 drop to the inside of each wrist.
Apply 1-2 drops directly onto sprain or joints or bottom of feet.
For sinusitis, apply 1-2 drops to the palm of hand, briefly touch palms together then cup over nose and mouth; breathe in deeply through the nose and out the mouth, 10x.

Inhalation:
May be inhaled or diffused: mentally stimulating, physically invigorating

Ingestion:
Ginger Oil from YLEO has GRAS designation advising it is safe to eat.
It can be added to food or drink.
- *Only Essential Oils with a GRAS designation should be ingested.*
    (Generally Regarded as Safe to Eat)

Essential Oil of Helichrysum (Helichrysum italicum)
Action:
Anticoagulant, dissolves hematomas (blood clots), mucolytic (breaks up mucus), expectorant, antispasmodic (relieves

spasms), reduces scar tissue, stimulates liver, chelates chemicals from the body

Uses:
For hematoma (swelling or blood-filled tumor), bleeding, arteriosclerosis, arrhythmia, thrombosis, phlebitis, varicose veins, skin conditions, scar tissue

Used by European researchers for skin conditions including eczema and psoriasis, and for regenerating tissue and for improving circulation.

Application:
Apply 1-2 drops to the target area.

Essential Oil of Lavender (Lavandula angustifolia)
Action:
Antitumoral, antiseptic, analgesic (relieves pain), anti-inflammatory, anticonvulsant, mild sedative, skin tissue regeneration, wound healing

History:
In 1910, Scientist Rene Gattefosse first discovered Lavender's skin regeneration properties and ability to expedite wound healing when he severely burned his hands in a laboratory explosion. He wrote the following description of the event in his book *Aromatherapy*: *"Both of my hands were literally aflame, covered in burning substances. Then, both my hands were covered in rapidly developing gas gangrene. But just one rinse with the Lavender Oil immediately stopped the gasification of the skin tissue. This treatment was followed by sweating and healing began the next day." (Gattefosse, 1937)*

Only a very severe burn would lead to gas gangrene which is a life-threatening condition. Gatefosse documented that the *Lavender Oil immediately relieved the pain, stopped this severe infection and quickly healed the burn without scarring.*
Essential Oils Desk Reference. (2000). *Essential Science Publishing.*

Dr. Jean Valnet successfully used Lavender Oil on wounded soldiers for its antibacterial and wound healing properties. Two of his students, Dr. Paul Belaiche and Dr. Jean Claude Lapray expanded his work. They clinically investigated the antiviral, antibacterial, antifungal and antiseptic properties of Lavender and many other essential Oils. Lavender Oil is still listed in the *British Pharmacopoeia.*

Larrondo, J.V., et al. (1995). *Microbios.*

Guillemain, J., et al. (1989). *Ann Pharm Fr.*

Kim, H.M., et al. (1995). *J Pharm Pharmacol.*

Uses:
Burns, cuts, bruises, wounds, skin care, asthma, bronchitis, convulsions, depression, heart palpitations, hives, insect bites, tumors, acne, dermatitis, rashes, eczema, psoriasis, laryngitis, abscesses, nervous, tension, insomnia

Application:
Apply 1-2 drops directly to burn, wounds, bruises, sore muscles, insect bites.
May be applied to throat glands, armpits, on sternum, on wrists on temples, or on the bottom of the feet.
Can 1 drop to face creams to improve complexion.
Can apply 4-5 drops along the spine and spread briefly with one fingertip.

Do not spread oil with the palm of your hand as oil will absorb into your hand.

Inhalation:
May be inhaled or diffused: both physically and emotionally calming, relaxing and balancing

Essential Oil of Lemon (Citrus limon)
Action:
Disinfectant, anti-infectious, antibacterial, antiseptic, antiviral, improves microcirculation, promotes white blood cell formation, improves immune function

Dr. Jean Valnet discovered that the vaporized essence of Lemon Oil can kill Meningococcus bacteria in 15 minutes, Typhoid bacilli in 1 hour, Staphylococcus aureus in 2 hours and Pneumococcus bacteria within 3 hours. He further confirmed that just a 0.2% solution of Lemon Oil can kill Diphtheria bacteria in 20 minutes.
Lemon Oil was widely used in hospitals in England as a disinfectant.

Uses:
Warts, moles, shingles, herpes, malaria, parasites, throat infections, varicose veins, to improve circulation.

Application:
Apply 4-5 drops along the spine and spread briefly with 1 fingertip.
Apply 2 drops to the bottom of the feet each morning as a preventative.
To shrink warts, moles or cysts: apply 1 drop of Lemon + 1 drop of Frankincense.

For cough, apply 1-2 drops onto the sternum and on spine between shoulder blades.

Add 20 drops to a spray bottle of filtered water and use it to disinfect surfaces.

Use this spray mixture to disinfect children's toys while also keeping children calm and focused.

It is safe to add several drops to the bath water of small children for a calming effect.

Inhalation:

May be inhaled or diffused: disinfects the air, stimulates mental clarity, physically invigorating and warming

Ingestion:

Lemon Oil from YLEO has *GRAS designation* advising it is safe to eat.

It may be added to food or drink.

- *Only Essential Oils with a GRAS designation should be ingested.*
   (Generally Regarded as Safe to Eat)

Essential Oil of Lemongrass (Cymbopogon flexuosus)

Action:

Helps to regenerate connective tissue and ligaments, dilates blood vessels, strengthens vascular walls, promotes lymph flow, anti-inflammatory, antifungal, antibacterial, supports digestion and is sedative.

Pattnaik, S., et al. (1996). *Microbios.* Lorenzetti, B.B, et al. (1991). *J Ethnopharmacol.*

Elsom, C.E., et al. (1989). *Lipids.*

Uses:

Aids in tissue regeneration of injured ligaments and tendons, swelling, sprains, respiratory infections, ringworm, improves microcirculation circulation.

Traditional uses were for purification of the body and digestive aid.

Clinical studies published in *Phytotherapy Research* records powerful antifungal properties of Lemongrass when applied topically.

Application:
Apply 2-3 drops directly onto swelling, sprain, injured tendon, ligament fungal infected or target area.

Inhalation:
May be inhaled directly or diffused: brings awareness and purification.

Essential Oil of Marjoram (Origanum majorana)
Action:
Soothes muscle, tones parasympathetic nervous system, helps to regulate blood pressure, supports respiratory system, dilates blood vessels, antibacterial, antiviral, anti-infectious

Uses:
Relaxes muscles, relieves anxiety, nervous tension, respiratory infections, fungal and viral infections, ringworm, shingles, muscle spasms, fluid retention, muscle spasms, cramps, sprains

History:
Traditionally, Marjoram was known as the *"Herb of Happiness"* to the Roman and as *"Joy of the Mountains"* to the Greeks. It was believed to increase longevity.

Application:
Apply 1-2 drops directly to the target area, sore or injured muscles.

Apply 1-2 drops to back of neck and between shoulder blades for tension headaches.

Can be added to coconut oil or almond oil to make a soothing massage oil.

Inhalation:
Can be directly inhaled or diffused for calming, to calm nerves.

Essential Oil of Melaleuca Alternifolia:

Action:
Antibacterial against large spectrum of gram positive and gram-negative bacteria, antifungal, antiviral, antiparasitic, antiseptic, anti-infectious, anti-inflammatory, immunostimulant (stimulates immune system), cardiotonic (supports heart function), neurotonic (supports nerves)

Hammer, K.A., et al. (1999). *Antimicrobial Agents Chemotherapy.*

Concha, J.M., et al. (1998). *J Am Podiatr Med Assoc.*

Syed, T.A., et al. (1999). *Trop Med Int Health.*

Uses:
Cold sores (Herpes simplex 1), shingles, athlete's foot, fungal infections, gum infections, respiratory infections, tonsillitis, thrush, candida

Application:
Apply 1 drop to the target area.

Apply 1 drop directly onto fever blisters, cold sores, nail fungus or nail infections.

Can be added to coconut oil to make foot massage cream for athlete's feet for fungal infection.

- *This is a strong oil.*
- Over-applying may cause itching. If so, apply coconut oil or olive oil to affected area

Inhalation:

May be diffused to cleanse and disinfects the air

Essential Oil of Myrrh Oil (Commiphora myrrha)

Action:

Anti-infectious, antiviral, antiparasitic, anti-inflammatory, relieves skin conditions, antihyperthyroid, supports immune system, laryngitis

Dolara, P., et al. (1996). *Nature.*
Al-Awadi, F.M., et al. (1987). *Acta Diabetol Lat.*
Michie, C.A., et al. (1991). *J R Soc Med.*

Uses:

Eczema, psoriasis, athlete's foot, fungal infections, hemorrhoids, dermatitis, ringworm, sore throat, chapped and cracked skin, wounds

History:

In Arabia, Myrrh was traditionally used for many skin conditions including dry cracked skin and wrinkles. Myrrh has one of the highest levels of *Sesquiterpenes,* a compound which has powerful effects on the brain, including the hypothalamus, pituitary (the master glands), and the amygdala (the seat of emotions).

Application:
Apply 1 drop to each throat gland or 2 drops to the sternum.
Apply 1-2 drops topically, or can add to coconut or almond oil to spread over a large area.
Can add 1 drop to face cream and apply before bed.
This oil is very thick and rich.

Inhalation:
May be directly inhaled by putting 1 drop into each palm, touching palms together briefly, cup palms over nose and mouth and breath in deeply, through the nose and out mouth.

Essential Oil of Oregano (Origanum compactum)
Action:
Powerful anti-infectious agent for respiratory, intestines, nerves blood and lymphatics with large spectrum action against bacteria, mycobacteria, fungus, virus, parasites, general tonic and immune stimulant

Uses:
Asthma, bronchitis, pulmonary tuberculous, whooping cough, respiratory infections, viral and bacterial pneumonia

Application:
Apply 1-2 drops under the ball and heel of feet, where skin is the thickest.

Caution: Oregano is a very strong oil!
- DO NOT APPLY DIRECTLY TO BODY UNDILUTED (except to ball and heel of feet where skin is thickest)
- Can be diluted with coconut oil or almond oil

- If itching occurs from overapplication, apply coconut oil, almond oil or olive oil over the area for relief. *DO NOT USE water, which only spreads the oil.*

Inhalation:
Can be diffused to disinfect air

Ingestion:
Oregano Oil from YLEO has GRAS designation advising it is safe to eat.
Can be used for cooking or added to food or drink.
- *Only Essential Oils with a GRAS designation should be ingested.*
   (Generally Regarded as Safe to Eat)

Essential Oil of Peppermint (Mentha piperita)
Action:
Reduces fever, anticarcinogenic, anti-acid, digestive aid, expels worms, decongestant, anti-infectious, antibacterial, antifungal, mucolytic (breaks up mucus), stimulant, expectorant, cardiotonic, anti-inflammatory for intestinal and urinary tract, stimulates mental clarity and focus.
   Gobel, H., et al. (1994). *Cephalalgia.*

Uses:
Asthma, bronchitis, diarrhea, indigestion, acid reflux, reduces fever, hot flashes, headaches, motion sickness, nausea, food poisoning, morning sickness, nerve regeneration, elevates sensory system

History:

Peppermint Oil is one of the oldest and most highly regarded Essential Oil. Dr. Jean Valnet performed extensive research on the beneficial effects of Peppermint Oil on the liver and respiratory system. It also stimulates an impaired sense of taste and smell. Dr. Dember of the University of Cincinnati confirms Peppermint Oils ability to increase concentration and mental accuracy. Dr. Alan Hirsch discovered Peppermint's ability to directly affect the brain's satiety center (the ventromedial nucleus of the hypothalamus) which triggers a sense of fullness after meals.

Application:
May apple 1 drops directly to temples for headache or to back of neck for a headache.
May put 1 drop on back of tongue for indigestion or for mental clarity and alertness.
May put 1 drop in a glass of water and drink with straw for acid reflux or indigestion.

Inhalation:
To clear sinuses, may be directly inhaled by putting 1-2 drops in each palm, touching palms briefly together, cupping hands over nose and mouth, then breathing deeply through nose and out mouth, 10x.
May be diffused to disinfect the air and to invigorate the mind and body.

Ingestion:
Peppermint Oil from YLEO has GRAS designation advising it is safe to eat.
It may be added to food or drink.
- *Only Essential Oils with a GRAS designation should be ingested.*

(Generally Regarded as Safe to Eat)

Roman Chamomile (Chamaemelum nobile)

Action:
Aids in skin regeneration, antispasmodic, antiparasitic, anti-inflammatory, antidepressant, emmenagogue (supports menstrual flow), calming
   Kennedy, A. (2016). *Essential Oils.*

Uses:
Boils, increases ability to regenerate skin tissue, aids liver in discharging toxins, improves insomnia, depression and nervous tension, restless legs, skin conditions, dermatitis, acne, eczema, reduces irritability and nervousness

History:
Traditionally, Roman Chamomile has been used for centuries for its calming properties and to relieve toothaches. It is also used in Europe for skin rejuvenation and regeneration.
   Essential Oils Desk Reference. (2000). *Essential Science.*

Application:
Apply 1-2 drops to the target area.
Apply 1-2 drops directly onto boils.
Apply to the bottom of feet, on ankles and on wrists for calming.
Apply 3-5 drops along the spine and spread briefly with one fingertip.
Must be added to carrier oil or cream if used on the face. Scent is strong.

Inhalation:
Can be inhaled or diffused for relaxing and calming effects.

Essential Oil of Rose (Rosa damascena)
Action:
Anti-inflammatory, anti-depressant, antiseptic, anti-viral, skin tonic, reduces scarring, skin tonic, balances and elevates mind, aphrodisiac
   Kennedy, A. (2016). *Essential Oils.*
   Sysoev, N.P. (1991). *Stomatologia.*
   Mahmood, N., et al. (1996). *Biochem Biophys*
      Res Commun.

Uses:
Broken capillaries, eczema, skin tonic, scarring, skin disorders and wrinkles, depression, migraines, nervous tension, menstrual problems

History:
For thousands of years, Essential Oil of Rose has been used for healing and beautification of the skin. Reputedly, the Arab Physician, Avicenna, was the first to distill Rose Oil. He even authored a book on its many healing properties.

Application:
May apply 1-2 drops to the target area.
Dilute with coconut, almond oil or aloe for use on face Add 1 drop to face cream. Scent is very strong.

Inhalation:
May be inhaled or diffused for mental balance and harmony.

Rich in Sesquiterpenes, Rose Oil has a rich intoxicating, aphrodisiac-like scent that balances and elevates the mind and is stimulating to the body.
Rose Oil has one of the highest Frequencies of all the Essential Oils, 320 Hz.

Essential Oil of Sandalwood (Santalum album)
Action:
Sandalwood supports nerves, circulation and brain function. High in Sesquiterpenes, Sandalwood, like Frankincense, has been extensively researched for its ability to stimulate the Pineal gland, the Pituitary gland and the limbic region of the brain, the center of emotions. The Pituitary gland is the master gland of hormone production. The Pineal gland is responsible for the release of Melatonin, a powerful neurotransmitter which induces deep sleep.
Essential Oils Desk Reference. (2000). Essential Science.

Uses:
Herpes simplex 1 and 2, urinary tract infections, acne, pulmonary infections,menstrual problems, meditation, nervous tension, skin infections, antiviral
   Benencia, F., et al. (1999). *Phytomedicine.*
   Dwiveda, C., et al. (1997). *Eur J Cancer Prev.*

History:
Traditionally, Sandalwood has been used for centuries in Ayurvedic medicine for skin revitalization and for meditation.

Application:
Apply 1-2 drops to the back of the neck, temples, wrists, behind ears.

Can be added to coconut oil or almond oil to make massage cream Can add 1 drop to face cream.

Inhalation:
May be inhaled or diffused for relaxing or enhancing deep sleep.

Spikenard (Nardostachys jatamansi)
Action:
Antibacterial, antifungal, anti-inflammatory, skin tonic, improves circulation

Dietrich Gumbel, Ph.D. affirms that Spikenard strengthens the heart and the circulatory system.

Uses:
Staph infections, insomnia, rashes, stress, tension, nourish skin

History:
Traditionally, Spikenard was highly regarded in India as a perfume, medical herb and skin tonic. It was one of the most precious oils used in ancient times, used by Kings and priests. It is recorded in the Bible that Spikenard was used by Mary Magdalene to anoint the feet of Jesus.

Application:
Apply 1 drop to the target area.
Apply 1-2 drops directly onto Staph infection.
May apply 1-2 drops over the heart or on abdomen.

Inhalation:
May be inhaled for relaxing and soothing effect

Essential Oils Desk Reference. (2000). *Essential Science.*

Vetiver (Vetiveria zizanioides)
Action:
Antiseptic, antispasmodic, anti-inflammatory, calms nervous system, supports production of red corpuscles, skin tonic

Uses:
Arthritis, rheumatism, insomnia, depression, anxiety, anger, skin tonic

Application:
Apply 1-2 drops to the target area
Add 1 drop to face cream.
Add 1 drop to coconut oil or almond oil for body or face treatment
Add several drops to carrier oil for a soothing massage.

Inhalation:
May be inhaled or diffused. Vetiver has an earthy, rich fragrance which promotes psychological grounding, calming and stress recovery.
   Kennedy, A. (2016). *EssentialOils.*

Ylang Ylang (Cananga odorata)
Action:
Antispasmodic, helps balance blood pressure, supports regular heartbeat, antidepressant, calming

Uses:
Palpitations, high blood pressure, anxiety, depression, mental fatigue, hair thinning, insomnia, impotence, rapid breathing, shock

History:
Heralded as an aphrodisiac, Ylang Ylang's rich scent has traditionally been used to perfume the bed of newlywed couples on their wedding night. It was also used to promote thick, lustrous, healthy hair.

Application:
Apply 2 drops on the sternum as a heart tonic.
Apply 1 drop to wrists and behind the ears as perfume.
Apply 1-2 drops below navel or to inner thigh crease to support sexual stimulation.

Inhalation:
Can be inhaled or diffused.
The rich scent of Ylang Ylang influences sexual energy while also promoting calm, joy and peace.

GENERAL PRECAUTIONS:

- *NEVER PUT ANY ESSENTIAL OIL INTO THE EYE OR EAR.*

- *If it gets into your eye, simply flush with coconut oil, olive oil or baby oil.*
  NEVER USE WATER which only spreads the oils and will not relieve the burning.

- *If you repeatedly over-apply an oil directly to the skin, it may start to itch.*
  Spread Coconut Oil, Almond Oil or Olive Oil over the affected area for relief. NOT WATER.

- *DO NOT put Frankincense on a burn.*
- *Remember, with Essential Oils "Less is More."*

TESTIMONIALS (the fun part)...
Severe Burn Healed...

I began using Essential Oils around 1990, when I was introduced to them by my Chinese masseuse, Chu-Chu. She informed me that Essential Oils had the unique ability to heal, prevent infection and bring oxygen and strength to the body overall. She advised that her family had been successfully using them for generations. I was in.

The first test came hard and fast. I had left a curling iron on all night. This was a very old curling iron, which did not have a heat controlling element in it. To be clear, the longer it was left on, the hotter it got. The next morning, thinking it was unplugged, I grasped the scorching hot curling iron by its chrome barrel instead of by the handle. The excruciating pain seared through my hand in seconds. The iron was so hot that the flesh on my palm and fingers melted and stuck to it. The burn was severe. I shook my hand loose and had a substantial meltdown. I needed to work that night and I needed the use of both my hands. The pain was horrible and I couldn't even close my hand as the burned flesh was so stiff, it felt like the skin was plastic.

I had recently purchased therapeutic grade *Lavender Oil*, which I studied was the best oil for a burn. I quickly put a few drops on my palm and fingers. I waited 5 minutes and put a few more drops. I waited 10 minutes and did it a third time. I was shocked and delighted to see that my pain disappeared almost completely after the third application, but what happened next was remarkable.

125

My hand did NOT even blister!...not later; not that night; not ever.

I had full use of it by evening and was able to go to work without the hindrance of pain, blistering or even stiffness.

I proceeded to learn all I could about these incredible oils, and I started using them on myself and my family, from that day on.

Mother's Shingles Healed...

Three years in a row, my Mother had contracted a severe case of Shingles all over her forehead, over her right eye and on her scalp. This always occurred right after she received a flu shot. She advised it caused a painful, burning sensation. This year, the doctor prescribed for her a $200 prescription called *Vioxx. This prescription not only did nothing to the Shingles but caused my mother to have immediate and horrible side effects including a distended abdomen, severe joint pain, inability to sleep* and overall malaise. It was clear to me that her body was saying *NO!*

My research confirmed that Shingles was a virus, actually a form of the Chicken Pox virus. I informed my Mother that no prescription can kill a virus. I proceeded to call the *Pharmacist who confirmed exactly that.* I then took that prescription and flushed it down the toilet.

Researching which Essential Oils would be most effective for Shingles, I chose to use what I called my "CLOM" Recipe: Clove, Lavender, Oregano and Melaleuca Essential Oils. I put a drop of each oil onto Mothers affected area 4 times a day. Each day, her symptoms visibly improved. *Within 7 days, they were gone.*

On day 9, my Mother's doctor called to check on her. She told him, *"I'm all better."* He replied, *"That's impossible!"*

His response confirmed to me that he knew all along that his prescription couldn't and wouldn't help her. He insisted that she come to his office so he could see for himself. He was astonished to see that anyone could be cured of such a bad case of Shingles in less than a week. He asked her to write down exactly what I had used on her. When he realized I used Essential Oils to heal her, he advised he was restricted from prescribing this to any of his patients, regardless of how well it works.

Mother never had another Shingles outbreak, ever.

- *Please Note:*
  Years later, a class action suit was generated against the makers of Vioxx as it was revealed that this drug caused heart attacks and strokes in many of its users. My Mother could have been one of those victims.

Cousin's Shingles Healed...

My cousin Shannon also contracted a bad case of shingles. The sores covered her right ribcage and half of her back. It was very painful for her. I gave her the same *"CLOM"* recipe that I used on Mother: *Essential Oils of Clove, Lavender, Oregano and Melaleuca.* I had her apply 1-2 drops of each oil to the infected area 4 times a day.

Success was ours in under two weeks. Her shingles healed and never returned.

Acid Reflux...

My Mother suffered from chronic acid reflux so severe that it began to erode her esophagus. The doctor gave her *Prilosec* to take. This caused her stomach to be filled with gas and made her constantly bloated. So, one day I tried putting a drop of *Essential Oil of Peppermint* into her drinking water. I made her drink it with a straw because oil floats and the Peppermint Oil may feel too strong against her lips. Mother took three sips. She was walking out of the kitchen with the glass in her hand when suddenly her eyes just flew wide open in surprise. She stopped in her tracks and declared, *"It's gone!…the burning is gone!"* This took less than 2 minutes.

That day, she stopped using everything except the Peppermint Oil for her acid reflux and was delighted with the successful results.

The Kindergarten Class (one of my favorite stories)...

In September of 1999, my baby girl was starting Kindergarten. A week later, her Teacher Judy advised that one student in the adjoining classroom had viral pneumonia, and that it was spreading through the classrooms. I quickly brought to school a large spray bottle filled with a mixture of filtered water with 30 drops of *therapeutic grade Essential Oil of Lemon. Lemon Oil is highly anti-viral.*

I instructed the Teacher to spray the desks of the students every morning and let it air dry. This way, the scent of the Lemon oil would be breathed in by each student sitting at their desk and would protect them from becoming infected. *I also gave her a diffuser filled with Lemon Oil to disinfect the air in the classroom. The results were remarkable!*

The Teacher was astonished that not only did no child in her classroom contract pneumonia, but in fact NONE of her 25 students got sick AT ALL for the next 7 months! She confirmed that in her 20 years of teaching 5-year-olds it has never happened that none of them got sick in almost an entire school year. She also thanked me for preserving her own health, as this was the first time she had not caught the usual continuous bouts of sickness from her students.

Lastly, the Teacher rejoiced in a very special *"Bonus"* *from the Lemon Oil.* She confirmed that breathing in the Lemon Oil caused her students to become *"very focused, calm and well-behaved, even through their Halloween candy eating!"* All the other Kindergarten Teachers asked her what was her secret for keeping a classroom of 5-year-olds so well behaved? She told them, *"Essential Oil of Lemon."*

A short time later, the other Kindergarten Teachers had diffusers and spray bottles of *Lemon Oil* in their classrooms, creating a calm, germ free, healthy learning environment for all.

- *Remember, I previously told you how Dr. Gary Young put a cotton ball with Lemon Oil in 1 nostril of an ADHD child, and it balanced that child's brain waves in 10 seconds. Lemon Oil has a safe, gentle yet profound effect on calming brain waves, especially in children, while also protecting them against sickness.*

Pilonidal Cyst Healed...

My friend Joan had a large Pilonidal Cyst right over her coccyx bone (tailbone). I had one many years ago and I can attest to how painful they are. Joan advised that *this cyst recurs every year,* and that she is forced to go to the doctor to have it lanced (sliced open) to scoop out all the pus. She had yet again scheduled an appointment to have this done.

I asked her to try using Essential Oils on her cyst this time, before having her procedure. I advised her to put a drop of *Frankincense Oil plus a drop of Lemon Oil* 4 times a day directly into the cyst. She was desperate to find a new solution.

Joan was astonished to see that her annual cyst started to shrink more and more each day, until it just

129

disappeared. It just melted completely away within 2 weeks. She called her doctor to cancel the procedure, advising her cyst was all gone. Her doctor asked what she used to heal the cyst. She told him that she applied *Essential Oils of Lemon and Frankincense.* He laughed and replied, *"Well then I'm not surprised the cyst is gone."* He was an Asian doctor who was very familiar with the healing power of Essential Oils.

Joan's "annual cyst" never returned.

Mole...

My same friend Joan had a large black mole on the side of her neck, as big as a pencil eraser. She had it for decades. I asked her to try putting a drop of *the Frankincense Oil and the Lemon Oil on it 4 times a day.* Remarkably, her mole just started shrinking. After a few weeks, that big mole ended up being just a flat pinkish mark that was hardly noticeable. The healing power of therapeutic Essential Oils is truly amazing.

Viral Pneumonia...

My good friend Lana advised me that her step-father Sam had been bedridden for a month with pneumonia. The doctors had given Sam round after round of antibiotics which had no effect on the pneumonia but only caused him to become weaker and weaker. I concluded that he had "viral pneumonia" since the antibiotics were clearly useless against it.

I gave Lana an *Essential Oil blend called "RC" from Young Living Essential Oils.* This blend is a powerful blend of 3 kinds of *Eucalyptus plus Myrtle, Pine, Spruce, Marjoram, Lavender, Cypress and Peppermint. These oils are a very potent treatment for chest, sinus and respiratory disorders.*

I advised Lana to put 3 drops on Sam's chest (sternum), 5-6 drops down his spine, 2 drops on the balls of his feet (this is the reflex point for the lungs). Lastly, I instructed that 3x a day, he put a few drops into his palms, touch his hands together briefly, cup over his nose and mouth, then breathe deeply in through the nose and out through the mouth, 10x.

On day THREE, Sam was up and out of bed! We were all astonished. Very quickly Sam's family committed to the belief that these therapeutic Essential Oils were an invaluable tool to keep on hand. Both then and now, I urge my family and friends not to be without them.

Asthma Attack Healed…

My friend Sharon had a 6-year-old boy named Victor who had severe asthma and allergies. Doctors had put Victor on steroids and steroid inhalers (nebulizers) which had little effect on his asthma, and appeared to have only inhibited his growth, as he was very small for his age.

One day, I went over to Sharon's house and saw her son on the couch having very labored breathing from his asthma. I noted he was also coughing continuously. I asked his mom if I could put some *RC* on him. *RC is a Young Living Essential Oil Blend of 10 powerful Essential Oils which is very effective against respiratory disorders.*

I proceeded to put the *RC* on the little boy's chest, feet, spine and underarms. I put a few drops onto my palms, cupped my hands over his nose and mouth and asked him to breathe in deeply 10 times. When finished, I spent the next 10 minutes telling his mom all about Essential Oils and how health promoting they are. *When, all of a sudden, we see Victor running, laughing, playing and roughly wrestling around with his older brother, without being winded and without coughing at all! In under 10 minutes, RC had that child off the couch* and behaving normally as a healthy little boy should. *My friend was amazed and frankly, I was too.*

The Croup Healed…

If you have ever heard anyone cough who has the croup, it is unforgettable.

A croup cough is a deeply disturbing "barking" sound, like a seal makes. It is even more disturbing when your young child has it. One night, I put my 2-year-old son to bed, and all was well. But in the middle of the night, I was awakened by a bout of coughing coming from his room. It was that deep, barking cough that told me immediately it was the croup.

The croup is the result of a virus which inflames the lungs. So, I ran to get my *RC Essential Oil blend, as well as my Frankincense and Lemon Oils*. I put 2 drops of each on his sternum, on his spine and under his feet.

He didn't cough again, not once, for the rest of the night. I oiled him once more before morning. He was perfectly fine the next day. The Essential Oils were completely successful in stopping the croup infection from growing inside his little lungs.

After I had my children, I made sure I kept Essential Oils on hand at all times. Because you never know when you or your child will start to be sick in the middle of the night. It is far easier to nip an infection in the bud, than to fight it once it is full-blown, and far less stressful on you and on your child.

Also, whenever we traveled, I carried Essential Oils in my handbag, suitcase, and in my carry-on luggage. My family and I literally went nowhere without bringing Essential Oils.

Fever Gone in Minutes…

My next-door neighbor, Mark, was home alone with

his 15-month-old son. The baby had a very high fever and Mark was distraught with worry. He brought the baby to me to see if I could help. The baby was wearing only a diaper and his skin was burning hot to the touch.

I knew that *Peppermint Oil was a fabulous fever reducer*. So, while Mark held the baby in his arms, I applied *Peppermint Oil* directly to the baby's spine, underarms and on the bottom of both feet. I then stepped back and, as usual, proceeded to sing the praises of Essential Oils to Mark, telling him of all their many benefits. Then, *all of a sudden…Mark's eyes flew open and he gasped!*

I said, *"what's the matter?"* Mark replied, *"He's COOL!…The baby's COOL!...His temperature just suddenly dropped, right here in my arms!"*

In 5 minutes, that baby's very high temperature just disappeared, just like that. It filled my heart to see the joy and relief in his father's face. It was the coolest thing ever…pardon the pun.

CAUTION: *Do NOT put Peppermint Oil near the throat or face of a baby or small child because the fumes are so strong. It would not harm them, but it would make them very uncomfortable and cause their little eyes to water. Therefore, notice I applied 1 drop of Peppermint Oil to this baby's back, underarms and bottom of feet and NOT to his neck or to his chest.*

Open Sores, Boils Healed…

Paul, the father of my good friend Rita, was suffering badly from a chronic outbreak of boils and open sores all over his body. He had worked with strong chemicals throughout his life. It appeared that now his body was reacting to an accumulated level of chemical poisoning. It was not enough to kill him; just enough to ruin his quality of life.

I consulted with Paul to assess his mental and physical condition. Both were dire. Paul advised new boils would break out every few days, in random places all over his body. He would get regular outbreaks even under his arms and around his waist so that he could not even comfortably wear his clothes. He said the boils *"were open, oozing holes in his flesh that were painful and so disgusting."* He said couldn't go out, and couldn't even stand looking at himself. Constantly, he was in pain. He had started drinking every day, in order to cope with this physical, mental burden. Finally, Paul admitted he was in complete despair, not wanting to go on living this kind of life, in pain and in constant dread of what new outbreak the next day would bring. He was at his wit's end. My heart went out to him.

I diligently dug through my Essential Oils research to find the most effective oil for healing boils and open sores. I came up with *Essential Oil of Roman Chamomile.*

I instructed Paul to simply apply ONE DROP of the Roman Chamomile on each of his existing sores and also wherever he feels a new one is coming. (He had advised he feels a burning sensation where a new sore is about to happen.) He called *THREE DAYS LATER* later, almost in tears. He jubilantly advised that wherever he put the *Roman Chamomile, that open sore would start to close the same day and heal up by the next day or two! Also, to his delight, when he feels a new boil coming, he puts the Roman Chamomile on that exact spot, and it stops that outbreak from happening. I was so thrilled for him!*

Just sharing some "Uncommon Knowledge" literally changed this man's life. I was, and I am still humbled and thankful to God for enabling me to share this wealth of health-

giving, life-changing knowledge to the blessing of all who will hear.

Hematoma Healed…

A hematoma is when blood pools under the skin, forming a swollen purplish lump, as a result of an injury to the wall of an underlying blood vessel.

One night, my rambunctious 3-year-old son came running full speed into my bedroom, in the dark. Well, of course, he smashed his forehead against one of my bedposts and fell backwards onto the floor screaming. I ran to him to find that a hematoma was forming before my very eyes. The space between his eyebrows was quickly filling with blood, so that a horrifying purple lump was protruding from his forehead, like a unicorn. I didn't have time to look up which Essential Oil to use, so I just grabbed the *"Daddy of all Essential Oils"….Frankincense.*

I quickly applied 2 drops to the blood bulge between his eyes. I waited 5 minutes and applied 2 more drops. I waited 10 minutes and did this a third time. What happened next was astonishing. I literally watched this huge purple lump *RECEDE* back into my son's forehead until it was FLAT. *It was as if someone hit the "rewind" button on a video.* Like a good Mother, I tried to appear calm in front of my son; but inside*, I was flipping. It's very hard not to use the word "miraculous" with these oils.*

I still get goosebumps whenever I tell this story.

Baby Teeth Knocked Out…

One fine day, my toddlers were playing in their room, jumping up and down on the bed. My daughter was 3 and my son was 2. Suddenly, my daughter came down onto the bed just as my son jumped up. His head hit her under her jaw, knocking out her four front bottom teeth. They were sticking straight out from her mouth at a 90-degree angle, yet somehow still attached to her gum by a prayer. Blood was everywhere. It was like a scene from a horror movie.

I ran and grabbed my *Essential Oil of Lavender* as I knew it was a great healer and that it was safe to put in her mouth (GRAS designation). I put some on my finger and rubbed it across her bottom bleeding gums. Then I took a warm wet cloth and gently pushed the teeth up and back, into their place, praying they would somehow reattach. As you know, baby teeth have no roots.

I then called the Pediatrician's medical emergency number. The Doctor advised that those 4 teeth *would NOT reattach* but, not to worry, because "they are just her baby teeth" and that her "second teeth" would come in eventually, to replace them...*well yeah, in 3 years!* I was *not* happy with that prognosis. I put more Lavender Oil on her gums before she went to bed and prayed for the best.

The next morning, my daughter's teeth were a bit wobbly but still in place. So, things were looking up. I put more lavender on her gums and waited.

By the end of the third day, all 4 teeth were firmly reattached. Not bleeding, not wobbly and not sore. I was so thankful that my sweet daughter didn't have to go 3 years with no bottom front teeth! Her doctor couldn't believe it. It was Lavender Oil to the rescue.

Fever Blisters, Cold Sores Healed...

Emma was a dear friend of ours who was plagued by cold sore outbreaks around her mouth all her adult life. Cold sores or fever blisters as they are sometimes called, are usually caused by the *herpes simplex 1 virus (HSV-1)*. A fever blister or cold sore is a visible symptom of the virus hijacking healthy cells. When Emma asked me what she could do to remedy this situation, I asked her to try putting a drop of Essential Oil of Melaleuca on each cold sore.

A few days later, Emma was thrilled to advise that, *not only did the Melaleuca Oil make the existing fever blisters disappear, but now if she feels one coming, she applies a drop to that area and the new fever blister does not emerge at all.*

The smallest victories in our health make the biggest difference in our life, don't they?

Gout Healed...

One morning, my good friend woke up with severe pain, swelling and redness in his big toe. I knew by the look of it and the pain level that it was the gout. Gout is caused by too much uric acid in the blood. I got to work researching the best Essential Oil to use. I chose *Geranium Oil.*

I had him put 2 drops on the big toe and toe joint 3 times that day. The very next day it was almost gone. By the third day, it was gone completely and never returned.

Ankle Injury...

And here I am with yet another story about my son. By now you have gathered that he was a bit of a *Dennis-the-Menace.* At age 5, his foot was caught between the car tire and the curb (don't ask). The foot turned bluish-black in minutes. Before taking him to the emergency room, I applied Essential Oils of Lemongrass, Cypress and Lavender to his foot, 3 times.

Before we even left for the hospital, the swelling in his foot had reduced to half, and the color of his skin went from blackish to light purple. Thankfully, we learned nothing was broken. By using Essential Oils treatment at home, his foot quickly and thoroughly healed without any residual pain or restrictions.

These are the times when you remind yourself of 2 things:
 1) Being a parent is NOT for the faint of heart.
 2) You must have Essential Oils on hand at all times
  for emergencies.

Knee Replacement Surgery...

Many years ago, my Dad had a knee replacement surgery at the age of 75.

After the surgery, Pop was sent to a rehab for physical therapy. Every day, I would go to visit him there and put *therapeutic grade Essential Oil of Lavender* directly onto his fresh incision. He was roommates with another patient who had the same surgery on the same day. *To the surgeon's surprise, Pop recovered twice as fast as his roommate.*

Pop also set a record at that rehab for being the first patient to be able to ride the stationary bike in the shortest time from date of surgery.

Another home run for Lavender Oil.

- *Only a Pure Therapeutic Grade Lavender Oil* is safe for open wounds.

Never Missed a Day of School from Sickness...

Believe it or not, my children have never missed a single day of school from sickness. All the many children in my neighborhood were sick about 2-3 times a month throughout the school year; but my children just never got sick.

One day neighbors converged upon me to ask, *"WHY are your kids never sick?"* I replied, *"Because I 'oil them' every morning and every night of their life."*

138

The Teachers at school always commented on how my children *smelled* when they came to school, saying some days they smelled like *lemons* (*RC Oil*) and other days they smelled like *apple pie* (*Thieves Oil*). I would apply RC on their throat glands every morning and some days I would put a drop of Thieves on their chest. After their bath and before bed, I put Lavender Oil on their chest and throat glands, and *Peace and Calm (YLEO blend)* on the inside of their wrists. Sometimes, I would put some Lavender drops in their bath water, making it like a heavenly scented, health spa treatment for my babies…and well…*they slept like babies.*

Caution:
Please do NOT put Thieves on a child's throat because it is a very strong oil blend and may cause them to itch. If this happens, put coconut oil, olive oil or baby oil over it and the itch will stop. *DO NOT USE WATER which only spreads the oil.*

Heart Palpitations…
I have had occasional heart palpitations since I was 17 years old. Exhaustion and low blood sugar triggered them. When they would occur, they could last for 3 hours and cause severe pain in my chest. I would be weak and debilitated until they stopped.

When I discovered Essential Oils, I discovered a final solution to this lifelong occurrence. When a palpitation hits me, I simply put a drop of *Frankincense Oil* inside my left elbow, on my chest. I also put 2 drops into my palms, cup them over my nose and mouth, and breathe it in through my nose deeply, and out through the mouth, 10 times.

In minutes the palpitations stop. Remember *Frankincense* is high is *Sesquiterpenes*, which is a component that crosses the blood-brain barrier. So the *Frankincense* has the ability to immediately balance the portion of the brain that governs heartbeat.

- *Please note:*
  This does NOT mean that Frankincense will correct a serious structural defect in your heart. You should see a cardiologist to ascertain the condition of your heart.

No Travel Sickness or Post Air-Travel Sickness…

Anyone who travels is well aware of the *post air-travel* cough, cold or sickness that often ensues about 2-3 days after a flight. Well, we traveled a lot. So I made sure that I oiled my husband, myself and the children before we boarded the plane, and also while we were on the *plane to ward off the multitude of germs that were airborne…while we were airborne.*

As a result, we never had post air travel sickness.

HDHD…

I had a friend whose daughter Amy had ADHD. Amy was 12 years old, yet could not even sleep through the night; nor could she sit very long in her seat at school. I asked her mother to put a few drops of pure Therapeutic Grade *Essential Oil of Lemon* on Amy's chest in the morning before school and at night before bed. I also asked her to put a few drops of the *Lemon Oil* onto some cotton balls and put them into a zip-lock bag. I instructed that Amy bring the ziplock bag to school to open it and just breathe in the Lemon Oil several times throughout the school day.

A few days later, my friend joyfully advised me that Amy was now sleeping all through the night. Also, her teacher actually called to ask, *"What are you giving Amy? Because she is suddenly staying in her seat all day!"* From a *simple choice came a major change in this child's life. Inhaling Essential Oil of Lemon.*

Remember: Lemon Oil is high in Sesquiterpenes, which is the component that crosses the blood-brain barrier to balance brain waves. Breathing it in through the nose causes it to travel immediately through the olfactory bulb, that is, it passes immediately from the nose to the brain, effectively balancing brain waves.

(Or you can just pretend it's Magic; because it sure feels like it ;)

Let's Wrap It Up…

By now you understand why I get so excited about sharing all these incredible healings with you. I can't promise you that Essential Oils will cure every single disorder under the sun, or even that you will have the exact same results I did, but I can affirm that *you will surely have a far greater chance of healing and health if you use them.*

I have been using YLEO therapeutic grade Essential Oils safely and successfully on my children, family and friends for almost 30 years. *Therapeutic Grade Essential Oils* are potent preventatives and healers which powerfully affect our body as well as our brain waves, emotions and behavior. Essential Oils can:

- Prevent and Heal infections by raising the body's Oxygen and Frequency.
- Travel throughout the body in minutes.
- Penetrate sick or dying cells.
- Expedite the healing of wounds
- Expedite healing injured muscles and ligaments
- Kill viruses, bacteria and fungi

- Balance erratic brain waves.
- Can be carried in your purse or your luggage as they do not need refrigeration.
- *Essential Oils have a longer shelf life than you or I have.*
- *It would be wise to have them on hand, BEFORE you need them.*

All the aforementioned testimonials resulted from my using Young Living Essential Oils, which are pure Therapeutic Grade.

- *It was safe to apply the YLEO Lavender Oil directly onto my father's raw incision because it is a pure therapeutic grade Essential Oil of Lavender and therefore was SAFE to apply to an open wound.*

- *An inferior Essential Oil will NOT render the same results and would be UNSAFE to apply to an open wound.*

NEXT ACTION:
"Follow the Recipe,"
...1,2,3...
1). Build and keep on hand your own Arsenal of Healing. I recommend starting with Lavender, RC, Peppermint, Lemon, and Thieves Oils. For overactive children, Peace & Calm blend is also great, especially at bedtime. blend.
There is so much power in these oils.

2). Apply a drop of RC or Lavender or Lemon Oil to throat glands and chest every morning; use Lavender or Peace &

Calm before bed. If you have children, it is KEY that you do this before school every day to avert common illness.

3). Keep at least RC and Lavender with you when you travel. There aren't many things worse than sick kids on vacation!

Product Information...
I am sure there are other Therapeutic Grade Essential Oils out there, but the one used in every one of my testimonials was Young Living Essential Oils (YLEO's).

- You can purchase *Young Living Essential Oils @ 800-371-3515.*
- You will be asked for a "Referral number" or "Member number."

Please Note:
You can use anyone's YLEO Member Number to place an order. You will receive your own number once you order. I am providing one here in case you don't have anyone else's to use.
Referral Member # 369730
Referral Member name: Linda Marie

- **I recommend YLEO simply because they have worked for me for 30 years.**

If you choose to use another brand of Essential Oil, **please be certain that they are pure Therapeutic Grade. I can't stress this enough.** *Otherwise, they will not have the amazing healing effects I have raved about in this chapter.*

The important thing is that you choose to protect your family's health by keeping some of these amazing Essential Oils on hand, because they are truly a Godsend.

Sir Francis Bacon, Lord Chancellor of England, once affirmed,
"Knowledge is Power."

And you should be feeling very powerful right now.

Chapter Three

YOUR BLOOD TYPE MAKES THE RULES
"Let Food be Your Medicine"

Let's talk about everyone's favorite pastime… *EATING.*

Enjoying good food is one of life's greatest gifts. With just a little applied knowledge, you can also use this gift to achieve and maintain a solid foundation of health and vitality. This chapter will be an eye-opener for many of you who may think all you have to do is not eat doughnuts and twinkies to get healthy. Although that's a great idea, remember in the preface of this book I advised that to achieve your best health**, you have to know what to eliminate from your daily life as well as what to add to it**.

This chapter will help you identify which foods are causing you inflammation, joint pain, thickened blood and weight gain; and no, they are not doughnuts or twinkies.

Dr. Peter D'Adamo is renowned for his exhaustive study of exactly how foods affect people with different blood types. For 40 years he, and eventually his son, studied the effects of foods on thousands of people with blood types A, B, O and AB. What he discovered and confirmed was that *the same food can have a beneficial effect on one blood type while having a very adverse effect on another blood type.*

145

This was a game changer for the world of nutrition, and in the lifelong pursuit of achieving optimal health.

In his best-selling book *Eat Right 4 Your Blood Type*, Dr. D'Adamo takes us down a fascinating path of the origin of blood types. Based on his 4 decade study, he painstakingly devised menus for each blood type, placing food groups into categories marked "Beneficial, Neutral and Avoid."

All the work is done for you. *You only have to go to the section with your blood type and learn which foods to avoid and which foods to add.* Surprisingly, there are only about a dozen "Top Avoid Foods" for each blood type. Learn them. Because this *Dirty Dozen* has the highest potential to negatively impact your blood, your joints and your health. Much of this chapter is based upon Dr. D'Adamo's life-changing discoveries.

Benefits of Eating Right for your Blood Type...

Through his extensive research, Dr. D'Adamo affirms that every food you eat reacts chemically with your blood type. Each blood type has a different reaction to foods. Discover here which foods are the *SuperStars* for your blood type and which foods are your *Dirty Dozen*. The core concept here is very simple:

- *Each blood type has a unique set of Beneficial and Avoid foods.*

- *Your Beneficial Foods are your SuperStars.* They are like natural medicine to your body. They promote health by reducing inflammation, regulating blood thickness, increasing energy, boosting your immune system, and promoting weight loss.

- *The Top Avoid Foods = Dirty Dozen. These foods promote ill-health.* They promote inflammation, thickened blood, suppress the immune function, cause weight gain, cell deterioration and promote disease.

- To achieve your highest health and vitality, you must simply *eat LESS of the Avoid foods and MORE of the Beneficial foods.*

Yes, it's that simple. The core level of your health will always begin and end with what you eat. The above 4 bullet points are the key to this entire chapter. They lay down an unshakeable concrete foundation for lifelong health.

What are Lectins…?
A Main Cause of Thick Blood and Blood Clots…
Lectins are a type of protein found in every food from plant to animal origin. *All foods contain lectins. This is NOT to be confused with Gluten.* Simply put, *lectins have different effects on different blood types*. Lectins can have *a complete opposite effect on* different blood types. For example, *kidney bean lectins can cause a great deal of inflammation and joint pain in blood in blood type O; yet they are beneficial to a blood type B.* This is just one small example of how you can be eating seemingly harmless food, yet your joints are getting stiffer and your blood is getting thicker month after month. *The dramatic effects of foods on different blood types is the foundation of Dr. D'Adamo's lifelong research, and it is the life-changing subject of this chapter.*

What Happens When You Eat "Avoid Foods"…

147

Avoid Foods are incompatible with your blood type. The lectins in your Avoid foods literally clump together or "glue together" your blood cells. This consequence is called *agglutination. This adverse reaction in your blood triggers common metabolic syndrome disorders, inflammation, thickened blood and weight gain.* When you continuously eat *Avoid Foods,* over time the lectins in that food will target an organ, joint or bodily system and will *begin to agglutinate (glue togethe*r) cells in that area causing acute inflammation and creating a host of health issues. Joint pain and arthritis are probably the best-known result of agglutination from eating incompatible/wrong foods for your blood type. All organs and systems of the body are susceptible to the adverse effects of incompatible food lectins.

The lectins from your Avoid foods can settle in any area of your body, where they have a *magnetic effect* on the surrounding cells in that region. They proceed to *clump together the healthy cells* in that area. Unrecognized by your immune system, your white cells "target these clumps for destruction," just as if they were invaders. In effect, *eating the wrong foods for your blood type often causes the body to attack itself (auto-immune disorders).*

- *The Lectins in your "Dirty Dozen"/Avoid Foods literally "clump your blood cells together" a little each day; for weeks; for months; for years.*

- *This causes progressive lifelong inflammation, thick blood, chronic joint pain, reduced organ function, suppressed thyroid and immune system, and weight gain and propensity for blood clots and stroke.*

"Tell Us About the Rabbi…!"
An Amazing Transformation of Health:

Dr. D'Adamo received a call from a New York Doctor regarding a patient in critical condition who was a Rabbi. This Rabbi was 73 years old and had a long history of poor health including poor circulation, swelling in his legs, and excruciating joint pain which escalated to the point of now preventing him from walking. He was on multiple injections of daily insulin yet his diabetes remained severe and uncontrollable.

When Dr. D'Adamo was contacted, the Rabbi had just suffered a massive stroke which left him partially paralyzed. The Rabbi was withered and bedridden. His only desire was to be able to walk again and to have enough strength to continue his work. He was a Blood Type B.

Dr. D. questioned the Rabbi's wife about what food he usually eats. The wife advised *that he eats the same food every day: chicken, bean paste, wheat noodles, and chicken fat. Every single one of these foods was an "Avoid Food" for a Blood Type B! Yet the wife confirmed that the unsuspecting Rabbi was eating all these foods not once a day, but TWICE a day, every day… for years.*

Over time, the lectins in these Avoid foods continued to agglutinate (glue together) the Rabbi's blood cells, thickening his blood, which most probably contributed to his blood clots and massive stroke. In a Blood Type B, the lectins in wheat are particularly obstructive to the effects of insulin, which rendered his diabetes uncontrollable. Lastly, for a Blood Type B, the lectins in chicken, corn and incompatible beans specifically attack the joints. Hence the Rabbi had very severe joint pain and very limited mobility. In short, this man was the perfect example of what dire health *consequences develop when you <u>regularly and continuously eat the wrong foods for your blood type</u>.*

> *The Rabbi was put on a Blood Type B diet, as follows:*
>> *Replace all chicken with turkey, fish, or lamb*
>> *Replace all wheat with rice, or millet*
>> *Replace all Adzuki beans, black beans, garbanzo and lentils with Kidney beans, Lima beans or Navy beans*

Within 6 weeks, the Rabbi was out of bed and exercising moderately. By 8 weeks, he was able to return to work. Within 6 months, he was switched to oral insulin instead of injectable, which was a major achievement after being on the injectable version for many years. For the first time, his diabetes was finally under control and he suffered no joint pain, inflammation or strokes to date, i.e., 6 years later.

D'Adamo, P. (1996). *Eat Right 4 Your Blood Type.*

How amazing is it that this man was resurrected from a dire state of health by 2 simple actions:
➢ *He "plugged the holes in his boat"*
   by eliminating his major top Avoid foods.
➢ *He "followed the recipe" by replacing these Avoid Foods with Highly Beneficial Foods for his blood type.*

The Missing Link…

Dr. D'Adamo declares he has finally *"identified the missing link in our comprehension of the process that leads either to the path of wellness or to the path of disease."* It's food. (D'Adamo,1996)

- After 4 decades of scientific proof, the beautiful truth is that we simply have to *match our food choices to our blood type.*

- *Let me advise here that whatever other healing modality you choose, if you do not eliminate at least the top 10 of your Avoid Foods from your diet, you are swimming against the tide of good health. After all, food is something we put into our bodies 3-5 times a day. So, eating the wrong foods for your blood type every day, will quickly blindside you with accumulated health consequences which become the lifelong mysterious cause of ill health.*

Blood Type is Your Genetic Inheritance and the Owner's Manual for Your Body…

Your Blood type is your cellular fingerprint. It has a genetic memory similar to your DNA. Your Blood type defines you more than your race or culture. Blood type is the key to the entire immune system, and thereby strongly defines your health profile. Your specific *Blood type dictates which foods you should be eating* and which foods you should be avoiding for optimal health. The main Blood types are: A, B, O, and AB.

Each Blood type has its own *antigens* which are the gatekeepers to your health. These *antigens* produce *antibodies* which attack any perceived threats to the body. When your blood detects an invader, it reacts by sending *antibodies* which attack the invader and literally glues their cells together by the *agglutination* process. Your body then produces white blood cells and hydrogen peroxide to destroy those enemy cells. *It's a fascinating protection mechanism!*

151

In Like manner, your blood type protects itself against other blood types entering the bloodstream, as they are also perceived as an invader. Your blood's "anti-other-blood-type-antibody" is so powerful that the agglutination process can be seen on a glass slide with the naked eye. *Your blood reacts in a very similar way when it detects incompatible food lectins in your blood.*

A Chemical Reaction Occurs between our Blood and the Food we Eat….

An extreme example of this reaction can be seen with a deadly chemical called *ricin.* Ricin is made from a toxic concentration of lectins from the castor bean. Once in the bloodstream, ricin causes *extreme agglutination* by gluing red blood cells into large clots which block the arteries and cause almost immediate death. *Please note, ricin was intentionally created as a weapon.* I am using it to show an *extreme example* of how, on a much lower level, incompatible food lectins can agglutinate your blood cells into clumps.

At the end of this chapter, you will find stunning testimonials from people of all ages who were healed of various disorders by simply eliminating the Avoid Foods for their blood type and adding the Beneficial Foods.

"Gimme the Short Version…"

- *Your Blood type is like the "Owner's Manual" that comes with your body.*
  Your body's reaction to the food that you eat is a genetic inheritance passed down from your blood type ancestors.

- *Beneficial Foods are like medicine. By adding your blood type's Beneficial Foods* to your diet, you will be strengthening your immune system and thyroid function, improving joint health, decreasing the likelihood of blood clots and promoting weight loss.

- *Avoid foods trigger a host of disorders.* Each time we eat foods that are incompatible with our blood type, the negative health consequences to our body accumulate slowly over time. Eating the top Avoid foods over the course of years and decades, promotes a lifetime of inflammation and ill health.

- By simply *eliminating your top Avoid Foods*, you will most likely *reverse and eliminate* a host of existing health problems. These include: cell damage, joint pain, thick blood, inflammation, suppressed organ functions, suppressed immune system, auto-immune disorders, suppressed thyroid function and weight gain.

How Do I Find Out My Blood type…?

For under $10, you can go to Amazon and order an *at-home blood typing kit*. It's very simple and takes minutes to do. Also, your blood type is identified if you donate blood.

What are My "Avoid Foods"…?
Each blood type has its own list of Avoid Foods.

Dr. D'Adamo's book *Eat Right 4 Your Blood Type* advises a complete list of blood type food menus. You can also buy a pocket-size book for your blood type which you can carry with you as you learn. It is less than 100 pages long.

For example, one pocket book is entitled, *Blood Type O, Food, Beverage and Supplement Lists* by Dr. Peter J. D'Adamo. On Amazon, you can find these pocket book versions for each blood type. I gave them to my entire family as stocking stuffers for Christmas one year.

…Well of course I did.

For your empowerment, I have extrapolated for you a *short list (an abridged version) of "Beneficial and Avoid Foods"* for each blood type, as follows:

BLOOD TYPE O:
"O" is for Oldest Blood Type…
- **Meat eater**
- **Hardy digestive tract.**
- **Overactive immune system**
- **Needs intense Physical Activity and protein for efficient metabolism**

Blood Type O is the oldest and most predominant of all Blood types. Comprising 80% of the population, it is the "Universal Donor" for all positive blood types. Genetics dictate a high protein diet with animal meats at the top of the list. *O's thrive on a high protein, high good fat diet.* This puts their body into slight *ketosis*, where the body metabolizes proteins and fats into *ketones*, a high-power cell fuel used in place of sugar. This is an optimal state for type O's, causing their muscles to be slightly acidic, healthy and charged for physical activity.

Diet...

Blood Type O's thrive on animal meats. As the original hunter/gatherers, their blood type demands high protein and exercise. Historically, they have strong stomach acids which are well adapted for the digestion of meats. Chemical-free organic meats are best. Wheat should be avoided, as the gluten in wheat inhibits their insulin metabolism. *Kidney bean, corn and lentils should be avoided* also, as they tend to cause joint pain, slower metabolism and muscle alkalinity for a Blood Type O. Muscle alkalinity in type O renders the muscles less charged for physical activity. Their Metabolism is optimized when their muscles are in a slightly acidic state. Type O's usually need additional iodine to fine tune thyroid function. This can be achieved by way of taking kelp supplements or by taking sublingual thyroid drops.

Stress...

Type O's have the ability to reverse the negative side effects of stress. Because this blood type has been ingrained with a "patterned alarm response," stress goes right into the muscle. This triggers an explosion of intense physical energy. When you encounter stress, the adrenal glands of your body take over. Type O's are built to release built up hormonal responses through intense physical exercise. Because the impact of the stress hormone cortisol is direct and physical, regular exercise is critical to the health of Blood type O's.

Personality Traits...

Blood Type O's carry the genetic memory for strength, endurance, daring and intuition. Type O's were a prime example of optimism, drive and confidence. They exhibit strong leadership qualities such as power and certainty. Great Britain's Queen Elizabeth II was a Blood type O.

THE SHORT VERSION OF FOODS FOR BLOOD TYPE O...

The following is a *quick glance list* of "Beneficial" foods that promote health and weight loss and "Avoid" foods that promote inflammation, ill health and weight gain for Blood Type O:

Major Beneficial Foods for Blood Type O:
Red Meat, Liver, Fish, Kelp, Iodized salt, Kale, Spinach, Sweet Potato, Broccoli, Flaxseed, Plums, Cherries, Blueberries, Bananas.

Major Avoid Foods for Blood Type O:
Corn, Wheat, Kidney beans, Navy beans, Lentils, Bacon, Ham, Pork, Cauliflower, White Potato, Honeydew, Oranges

The Key to Success...

- *The key action here is to eliminate all or most of the 12 Dirty Dozen Avoid Foods listed in the above Short Version as they are the most damaging for Blood Type O.*

- *Any additional Avoid Foods can be slowly replaced with Beneficial foods as your individual taste dictates. Eating Avoid Foods once in a while is not going to be nearly as detrimental as eating them every day or every week.*

- *Rule of thumb is that any food that is not listed in the Beneficial or Avoid List, is usually considered "Neutral."*

1. Highly Beneficial Meats and Poultry for Blood Type O:
Beef, Bufalo, Heart, Lamb, Liver, Veal, Venison
Avoid Meats & Poultry for Blood Type O:
Bacon, Ham, Pork, Turtle, Quail

2. Highly Beneficial Seafood for Blood type O:
Bass, Cod, Halibut, Perch, Pike, Red Snapper, Shad, Sole, Sturgeon, Swordfish, Tilefish, Rainbow Trout, Yellowtail
Avoid Seafood for Blood Type O:
Abalone, Barracuda, Catfish, Conch, Frog, Herring, Lox, Muskellunge, Octopus, Pollack, Squid

3. There is no Beneficial Dairy for Blood Type O.
Neutral Dairy for Blood Type O:
Butter, Eggs, Farmer's cheese, Feta, Ghee, Goat cheese, Mozzarella, Kefir, Milk, Yogurt
Avoid Dairy for Blood Type O:
American cheese, Blue cheese, Brie, Buttermilk, Camembert, Cheddar, Colby, Gouda, Gruyere, Jarlsberg, Muenster, Sour cream, Sherbert

4. Highly Beneficial Oils & Fats for Blood Type O:
Flaxseed oil, Olive oil, Rice bran oil
Avoid Oils & Fats for Blood Type O:
Castor oil, Corn oil, Cottonseed oil, Evening Primrose, Peanut oil, Safflower oil, Soy

5. Highly Beneficial Nuts & Seeds for Blood Type O:
Flaxseed, Pumpkin seeds, Walnuts
Avoid Nuts & Seeds for Blood Type O:
Beech, Brazil, Cashew, Chestnut, Litchi, Peanut, Pistachio, Poppy seeds, Sunflower seeds

6. Highly Beneficial Beans & Legumes for Blood Type O:
Adzuki beans, Black-Eyed peas
Avoid Beans & Legumes for Blood Type O:
Copper beans, Kidney beans, Lentils, Navy bean, Tamarind bean

7. Highly Beneficial Breads for Blood Type O:
Essene bread, (Ezekiel bread is *Neutral)*
Avoid Breads for Blood Type O:
Wheat, Corn, Matzo, Multi-grain, Pumpernickel, Wheat Bran, Whole Wheat

8. There are no Beneficial Grains for Blood Type O.
Neutral Grains for Blood Type O:
Buckwheat, Oat, Quinoa, Rice, Rye, Soba Noodles, Spelt
Avoid Grains for Blood Type O:
Barley, Bulgar, Couscous, Durum wheat flour, Graham flour, Semolina, Whole wheat flour, White flour

9. Highly Beneficial Vegetables for Blood Type O:
Artichoke, Beet greens, Broccoli, Chicory, Collard greens, Dandelion, Escarole, Ginger, Horseradish, Kale, Kelp, Kohlrabi, Lettuce, Okra, Onion, Parsley, Parsnip, Cayenne pepper, Sweet potato, Pumpkin, Seaweed, Spinach, Swiss Chard, Turnip
Avoid Vegetables for Blood Type O:
Alfalfa, Capers, Cauliflower, Corn, Cucumber, Leeks,

Shiitake mushrooms, Silver Dollar mushrooms, Mustard greens, Black olives, Pickles, Potatoes (blue, red, white), Rhubarb, Spirulina, Taro, Yucca

10. Highly Beneficial Fruits for Blood Type O:
Banana, Blueberry, Cherry, Fig, Guava, Mango, Plum, Prune
Avoid Fruits for Blood Type O:
Asian pear, Avocado, Blackberry, Cantaloupe, Coconut, Kiwi, Honeydew, Orange, Plantain, Tangerine

11. Highly Beneficial Juices for Blood Type O:
Black Cherry, Guava, Mango, Pineapple, Prune, Spinach
Avoid Juices for Blood Type O:
Aloe, Blackberry, Coconut milk, Cucumber, Orange, Tangerine

12. Highly Beneficial Spices for Blood Type O:
Carob, Curry, Dulse, Horseradish, Kelp, Parsley, Cayenne pepper, Turmeric
Avoid Spices for Blood Type O:
Acacia, Aspartame, Carrageenan, Cornstarch, Corn syrup, Fructose, Invert Sugar, Mace, Maltodextrin, MSG, Nutmeg, Black pepper, White pepper, Sucanat, Sucrose

13. Highly Beneficial Beverages for Blood Type O:
Club soda, Seltzer water, Green tea, Astragalus tea, Dandelion tea, Chickweed tea, Ginger tea, Mulberry tea, Sarsaparilla tea, Slippery Elm tea
Avoid Beverages for Blood Type O (abridged):
Alfalfa tea, Echinacea, Goldenseal, Red Clover, Rhubarb tea, St. John's Wort, Beer, Coffee, distilled Liquor, Soda, Black tea

Worth Repeating*:*

- *The key here is to at least eliminate all or most of the major Avoid Foods listed in the previously advised **Short Version,** as they are the most damaging for Blood Type O.*

BLOOD TYPE A:
"A" is for "Agrarian"...

- **Vegetarian**
- **Sensitive digestive tract**
- **Adapts well to environmental conditions**
- **Requires Agrarian Diet to stay lean and productive**

When farming and the cultivation of grains eclipsed the hunter/gatherer era, Blood Type A's quickly mutated from Blood Type O out of survival necessity. Blood Type A began to thrive in an agrarian/farming society, even becoming more resistant to infections due to environmental stress of increased population. Over time, their evolved mostly grain and vegetable diet caused them to lose the ability to efficiently digest red meats. Most dairy may also be poorly digested by Blood Type A. *They commonly have low stomach acid. This blood type thrives on vegetables and grains.*

- *Blood Type A's should eliminate all processed meats such as deli meats, cold cuts, ham and hotdogs which can promote stomach cancer in those with low stomach acid.*

Diet...

Type A's are born vegetarians. Forced by the necessity of migration, they have adapted to an agrarian

160

lifestyle. Type A's should limit their dairy intake, as it causes them to overproduce mucus. Tomatoes can irritate their stomach. Low stomach acid dictates eating very little if any red meat. An A thrives in slightly alkaline muscle tissue. This blood type needs to boost its protein intake with eggs, fish, peanuts, tofu and beans. Careful attention should be paid to maintaining proper levels of iron by way of eating blackstrap molasses or iron supplements. Lastly, because of the lack of red meat in this diet, a sublingual B-12 supplement would be wise.

Stress…

Type A's have the ability to reverse the negative effects of stress. Stress equates to type A in the form of an intellectual alarm. Their adrenaline response triggers anxiety, irritability and hyperactivity. This heightened sensitivity of their nervous system wears away at their immune system. A deep and prolonged state of stress is especially deleterious to the health of an A Blood Type. A's need to overcome stress via calming techniques, such as meditation, relaxation, deep breathing and focused stillness. Intense sports or exercise can exhaust the nervous system. Meditation, Tai Chi, Yoga or any practice that promotes calm and centering are the remedy to rescue type A's from the grip of stress.

Personality Traits…

Type A's are usually clever, cooperative, sensitive and passionate, all traits that were necessary to adapt to their changing environment and to meet the challenges of a new and complex life. However, this comes with the price of being "tightly wired." A's tend to have bottled up anxiety which can be managed by way of the above calming mechanisms.

161

THE SHORT VERSION OF FOODS FOR BLOOD TYPE A...

The following is a *quick glance list* of *"Beneficial Foods"* that promote health and vitality, and *"Avoid foods"* that promote inflammation, ill health and weight gain for Blood Type A:

Major Beneficial Foods for Blood Type A:

Fish, Vegetables, Soy foods, Pineapple, Lemon, Lentils, Black beans, Pinto Beans, Black-Eyed peas, Soybeans, Tofu, Peanuts, Flaxseed, Pumpkin seed

Major Avoid Foods for Blood Type A:

Bacon, Ham, Pork, Cold Cuts, Red Meat, Kidney beans, Lima beans, Navy Beans, Cashews, Pistachios, (abundance of) Wheat, Cabbage

The Key to Success...

- *The key action here is to eliminate all or most of the 12 Dirty Dozen Avoid Foods listed in the above Short Version as they are the most damaging for Blood Type A.*

- *Any additional Avoid Foods can be slowly replaced with Beneficial foods as your individual taste dictates. Eating Avoid Foods once in a while will not be nearly as detrimental as eating them every day or every week.*

- *Rule of thumb is that any food that is not listed in the Beneficial or Avoid List, is usually considered "Neutral."*

1. There are no Beneficial Meats or Poultry for Blood Type A.
 Neutral Meats for Blood Type A:
>Chicken, Cornish hen, Guinea hen, Ostrich, Turkey
Avoid Meats for Blood Type A:
>Bacon, Ham, Pork, Beef, Buffalo, Duck, Goose, Lamb, Liver, Pheasant, Quail, Rabbit, Sweetbreads, Turtle, Veal, Venison

2. Highly Beneficial Seafood for Blood Type A:
>Carp, Cod, Mackerel, Monkfish, Perch, Pollack, Red Snapper, Salmon, Sardine, Snail, Trout, Whitefish, Whiting
Avoid Seafood for Blood Type A (abridged):
>Anchovy, Barracuda, Bass, Bluefish, Catfish, Caviar, Calm, Conch, Crab, Crayfish, Eel, Flounder, Frog, Grouper, Haddock, Halibut, Herring, Lobster, Lox, Mussels, Oysters, Scallops, Shrimp, Squid

3. There is no Highly Beneficial Diary for Blood Type A.
 Neutral Dairy for Blood Type A:
>Eggs, Farmer's cheese, Feta, Ghee, Goat cheese, Kefir, Goat milk,
Mozzarella, Ricotta, Sour cream, Yogurt
 Avoid Dairy for Blood Type A (abridged):
>American, Blue cheese, Brie, Camembert, Cheddar, Colby, Cream cheese, Gouda, Gruyere, Jarlsberg, (pasteurized) Cow's milk, Monterey Jack cheese, Muenster cheese, Provolone, Sherbert

4. Highly Beneficial Oils & Fats for Blood Type A:
>Black Currant seed, Flaxseed, Olive, Walnut
 Avoid Oils & Fats for Blood Type A:
>Castor, Corn, Cottonseed, Peanut, Safflower

5. Highly Beneficial Nuts & Seeds for Blood Type A:
Flaxseed, Peanut, Peanut butter, Pumpkin seed, Walnut

Avoid Nuts & Seeds for Blood Type A:
Brazil, Cashew, Cashew butter, Pistachio

6. Highly Beneficial Beans & Legumes for Blood Type A:
Adzuki, Black, Black-Eyed peas, Stringbeans, Lentils, Pinto, Soybeans, Soy milk, Tofu

Avoid Beans & Legumes for Blood Type A:
Copper, Garbanzo, Kidney, Lima, Navy, Tamarind beans

7. Highly Beneficial Bread for Blood Type A:
Essene, Ezekiel, Soyflour

Avoid Bread for Blood Type A:
Matzo, Pumpernickel, Wheat Bran, Whole Wheat

8. Highly Beneficial Grain for Blood Type A:
Amaranth, Buckwheat, Oat, Rye, Soba, Soy flour, Kasha, Oatbran, Oatmeal

Avoid Grain for Blood Type A:
Cream of Wheat, Farina, Grape Nuts, Wheat Germ, Shredded Wheat, Wheat Bran

9. Highly Beneficial Vegetables for Blood Type A:
Alfalfa, Artichoke, Beet greens, Broccoli, Celery, Carrots, Chicory, Collard greens, Dandelion, Escarole, Garlic, Ginger, Kale, Leeks, Mushrooms, Parsley, Parsnip, Pumpkin, Spinach, Swiss Chard, Turnip

Avoid Vegetables for Blood Type A:
Cabbage, Capers, Chili Peppers, Eggplant, Juniper,

Shiitake mushrooms, Black olives, Cayenne pepper, Peppers (green, red, yellow), Potatoes (red, sweet, white, yellow), Rhubarb, Sauerkraut, Tomato, Yam, Yucca

10. Highly Beneficial Fruit for Blood Type A:

Apricot, Blackberry, Blueberry, Cherry, Cranberry, Fig, Grapefruit, Lemon, Lime, Pineapple, Prune

Avoid Fruit for Blood Type A:

Banana, Coconut, Mango, Honeydew melon, Orange, Papaya, Plantains, Tangerine

11. Highly Beneficial Juices for Blood Type A:

Aloe, Apricot, Blackberry, Carrot, Celery, Cherry, Grapefruit, Lemon, Lime, Pineapple, Prune, Spinach

Avoid Juices for Blood Type A:

Cabbage, Coconut milk, Mango, Orange, Papaya, Tangerine, Tomato

12. Highly Beneficial Spices for Blood Type A:

Barley Malt, Blackstrap molasses, Garlic, Ginger, Horseradish, Mustard, Parsley, Tamari, Turmeric

Avoid Spices for Blood Type A:

Acacia, Capers, Gelatin, Back pepper, Tamarind, Vinegar, Wintergreen

13. Highly Beneficial Beverages for Blood Type A:

Alfalfa, Astragalus, Burdock, Chamomile, Dandelion, Ginseng, Rose Hip, St. John's Wort, Slippery Elm teas, Coffee, Green tea, Red wine

Avoid Beverages for Blood Type A:

Catnip, Corn Silk, Goldenseal, Juniper, Red Clover, Rhubarb, Yellow Dock teas, Beer, distilled Liquor, Seltzer water, Club soda, Black tea.

Worth Repeating:
- *The key here is to at least eliminate all or most of the major Dirty Dozen Avoid Foods listed in the previously advised **Short Version,** as they are the most damaging for Blood Type A.*

BLOOD TYPE B:
"B" is for "Balanced"...
- *Dairy eater*
- *Strong immune system*
- *Tolerant digestive system*
- *Needs physical and mental activity for balance*

The diet for Blood Type B is somewhat of a melange of O and A blood type diets. That is, Blood Type B's can eat the best of the animal and vegetable kingdoms.
But, just like Type O, wheat, corn and lentils show down the metabolism of a Blood Type B. Blood type B's have a hardy immune system, often healing from common diseases which other blood types succumb to. However, they may be prone to auto-immune disorders. Choosing to eat a healthy blood type diet can greatly increase probability for a long healthy life for all blood types.

Diet...
Blood Type B is the assimilator. *They thrive on meats, most vegetables and a wide selection of dairy.* The inclusion of specific dairy foods in a type B diet actually balances their metabolism. However, *wheat lectins* attach to their insulin receptors prohibiting the insulin from attaching. To avoid weight gain and slowed metabolism, *B's should avoid wheat,*

corn, lentils and sesame seeds. Most nuts and seeds are not advised for B's, as the wrong ones interfere with insulin production (see the *Avoid* nuts).

- *Type B's should make a point of replacing all chicken with turkey, as chicken contains a strong agglutinating lectin in its muscle tissue which is detrimental to a Blood Type B. (Remember the Rabbi.)*

Stress…

Type B's response to stress is a balance between the nervous mental activity of type A and the physically aggressive response of type O. Type B's were both nomads and agrarians. B's usually confront stress well, and are well adapted for blending into unfamiliar situations. They maintain calm with moderate exercise that is not too physically intense.

Personality Traits…

Type B's are usually less confrontational than O's but more physically adaptive to stress hormones than A's. Type B's ancestral traits of flexibility and creativity were necessary for the early type B's to survive intermingling with new races and cultures. Typically, B's relate easily to different personality types, and are disinclined to challenge or confront. They maintain harmony by way of maintaining mental and physical balance.

THE SHORT VERSION OF FOODS FOR BLOOD TYPE B…

The following is a *quick glance list* of *"Beneficial Foods"* that promote health and weight loss, and *"Avoid Foods"* that promote inflammation, ill health and weight gain for Blood Type B:

Major Beneficial Foods for Blood Type B:

Meat, Liver, Fish, Eggs, Cottage cheese, Feta, Milk, Mozzarella, Ricotta, Yogurt, Walnuts, Green vegetables, Lentils, Kidney, Lima and Navy beans, Banana, Papaya, Pineapple, Plum, Grapes

Major Avoid Foods for Blood Type B:

Bacon, Ham, Pork, Chicken, Corn, Wheat, Lentils, Peanuts, Cashews, Black beans, Soybeans, Pinto Beans,

The Key to Success...

- *The key action here is to eliminate all or most of the 12 Dirty Dozen Avoid Foods listed in the above Short Version as they are the most damaging for Blood Type B.*

- *Any additional Avoid Foods can be slowly replaced with Beneficial foods as your individual taste dictates. Eating Avoid Foods once in a while is not going to be nearly as detrimental as eating them every day or every week.*

- *Rule of thumb is that any food that is not listed in the Beneficial or Avoid List, is usually considered "Neutral."*

1. Highly Beneficial Meats & Poultry for Blood Type B:

Goat, Lamb, Mutton, Rabbit, Venison (Beef is neutral)

Avoid Meats & Poultry for Blood Type B:

Bacon, Ham, Pork, Cornish hen, Chicken, Duck, Goose, Quail, Sweetbreads, Turtle

2. Highly Beneficial Seafood for Blood Type B:

Caviar, Cod, Flounder, Grouper, Haddock, Mackerel, Monkfish Perch, Salmon, Sardine, Shad Sole, Sturgeon

Avoid Seafood for Blood Type B:

Anchovy, Bass, Beluga, Butterfish, Clam, Conch, Crab, Crayfish, Eel

3. Highly Beneficial Dairy for Blood Type B:

Cottage cheese, Farmer's cheese, Feta cheese, Goat's cheese, Kefir, Milk, Mozzarella, Ricotta, Yogurt

Avoid Dairy for Blood Type B:

American cheese, Blue cheese, Ice cream, String cheese

4. Highly Beneficial Oils & Fats for Blood Type B:

Olive oil

Avoid Oils & Fats for Blood Type B:

Avocado, Canola, Castor, Corn, Cottonseed, Peanut, Safflower, Sesame, Soy, Sunflower

5. Highly Beneficial Nuts & Seeds for Blood Type B:

Black walnuts

Avoid Nuts & Seeds for Blood Type B:

Cashew, Filbert, Pistachio, Peanut, Peanut butter, Poppy, Pumpkin, Sesame seeds, Sunflower seeds

6. Highly Beneficial Beans & Legumes for Blood Type B:

Kidney beans, Lima beans, Navy beans

Avoid Beans & Legumes for Blood Type B (abridged):

Adzuki, Black, Black-Eyed peas, Garbanzo beans, Lentils, Pinto, Soybeans,

7. Highly Beneficial Bread for Blood Type B:
Ezekiel Bread, Oatbran, Brown rice, Spelt, Rice cakes
Avoid Bread for Blood Type B:
Amaranth, Buckwheat, Corn, Pumpernickel, Rye

8. Highly Beneficial Grains for Blood Type B:
Millet, Oat, Oatmeal, Rice, Spelt
Avoid Grains for Blood Type B:
Amaranth, Buckwheat, Corn, Grits, Rye, Tapioca, Wheat Bran, Wheat Germ, Pumpernickel

9. Highly Beneficial Vegetables for Blood Type B:
Beets, Beet greens, Broccoli, Brussel sprouts, Cabbage, Carrots, Cauliflower, Collard greens, Eggplant, Ginger, Kale, Mushroom, Parsley, Parsnip, Peppers, Sweet potatoes, Yams
Avoid Vegetables for Blood Type B:
Artichoke, Corn, Olive, Pumpkins, Radish, Rhubarb, Tomato

10. Highly Beneficial Fruits for Blood Type B:
Banana, Cranberry, Grapes, Papaya, Pineapple, Plum, Watermelon
Avoid Fruits for Blood Type B:
Avocado, Coconut, Melon, Pomegranate, Prickly pear, Starfruit

11. Highly Beneficial Juices for Blood Type B:
Beets greens, Cabbage, Cranberry, Papaya, Pineapple

Avoid Juices for Blood Type B:
 Coconut juice, Pomegranate, Tomato

12. Highly Beneficial Spices for Blood Type B:
 Curry, Ginger, Horseradish, Parsley, Pepper (cayenne*)*
Avoid Spices for Blood Type B (abridged):
        Acacia, Allspice, Aspartame, Cinnamon, Cornstarch Corn syrup, Dextrose, Maltodextrin, Gelatin, MSG, Pepper, Tapioca

13. Highly Beneficial Beverages for Blood Type B:
Green tea, Ginger, Ginseng, Licorice Root, Milk Thistle, Peppermint, Rose Hip
Avoid Beverages for Blood Type B (abridged):
Goldenseal, Guarana, Hops, Juniper, Red Clover, Skullcap, Stinging Nettle Root distilled Liquor, Seltzer water, Club soda

Worth Repeating:
- *The key action here is to at least eliminate all or most of the major Avoid Foods listed in the previously advised **Short Version**, as they are the most damaging for Blood Type B.*

BLOOD TYPE AB:
"AB" is a Blend of both A and B Blood Types…
- *Thrives on A and B Blood type diets*
- *Rarest of Blood Types*
- *Strong Immune System*
- *Adapts well to Changing Environment*

Blood Type AB is the newest of all blood types, rarely being found prior to 900 A.D. Less than 5% of the population has Blood Type AB. Their immune systems are enhanced due to the fact they have inherited the tolerance of both A and B types. AB's have the ability to produce more specific antibodies to microbial infections, which minimizes their chances of having allergies or autoimmune disease. AB is the *Universal Receiver.*

Diet…

AB's have a unique blend of some pluses and minuses of Blood Types A and B.

Although they can eat tomatoes, vegetables and dairy, they inherited the low stomach acid of type A's, dictating the elimination of red meat from their diet. *AB's should avoid Kidney beans, Lima beans, Corn, Buckwheat and Sesame seeds, which interfere with insulin metabolism,* just like in Type B's. Type AB's do not usually have a severe reaction to wheat gluten, but to keep metabolism at optimal level, wheat should be kept to a minimum in their daily diet. Wheat gluten causes AB's muscle tissue to become *acidic* and AB's need *slightly alkaline* muscles for efficient metabolism.

- *Blood type AB's should eliminate all processed meats such as bacon, deli meats, cold cuts, ham and hotdogs which can promote stomach cancer in those with low stomach acid.*

Stress…

AB's have inherited the ability to reverse the negative effects of stress. They exhibit the same stress pattern as Blood Type A. AB's react intellectually to the first "alarm stage" of stress. Their adrenally charged brain produces anxiety, irritability and hyperactivity. This heightened

172

sensitivity of the nervous system suppresses the immune system. Calming techniques such as deep breathing, meditation and Yoga can counter the negative effects of stress with centering and relaxation. AB's do not respond well to continuous confrontation. A deep and prolonged state of stress is especially deleterious to the health of an AB. Therefore, Tai Chi or any exercise that promotes calm and focus are the remedy to rescue type AB's from the grip of stress.

Personality Traits…

Type AB's are a merging of the edgy, sensitive type A with the balanced, centered type B. Blood type AB's rarely hold grudges and are usually very diplomatic in their words and in their approach to things. President John F. Kennedy was an AB.

THE SHORT VERSION OF FOODS FOR BLOOD TYPE AB…

The following is a *quick glance list* of *"Beneficial foods"* that promote health and weight loss and *"Avoid foods"* that promote inflammation, ill health and weight gain for Blood Type AB:

Major Beneficial Foods for Blood Type AB:

Seafood, Turkey, Cottage cheese, Mozzarella, Sour cream, Yogurt, Tofu, Green vegetables, Kelp, Pineapple

Major Avoid Foods for Blood Type AB:

Bacon, Ham, Pork, Chicken, Red meat, Black beans, Garbanzo beans, Kidney beans, Lima beans, Corn, Buckwheat, Banana

The Key to Success...

- *The key action here is to eliminate all or most of the 12 Dirty Dozen Avoid Foods listed in the above Short Version as they are the most damaging for Blood Type AB.*

- *Any additional Avoid Foods can be slowly replaced with Beneficial foods as your individual taste dictates. Eating Avoid Foods once in a while will not be nearly as detrimental as eating them every day or every week.*

- *Rule of thumb is that any food that is not listed in the Beneficial or Avoid List, is usually considered "Neutral."*

1. Highly Beneficial Meats and Poultry for Blood Type AB:

Turkey

Avoid Meats and Poultry for Blood Type AB:

Bacon, Ham, Pok, Beef, Buffalo, Chicken, Cornish hen, Duk, Goose Quail, Sweetbreads, Turtle, Veal, Venison

2. Highly Beneficial Seafood for Blood Type AB:

Cod, Grouper, Mackerel, Mahi Mahi, Monkfish, Pike, Red Snapper, Sailfish Salmon, Sardine, Shad, Snail, Escargot, Sturgeon, Tuna

Avoid Seafood for Blood Type AB:

Bass, Beluga, Clam, Conch, Crab, Eel, Flounder, Halibut, Herring, Lobster, Lox, Octopus, Oyster, Salmon Roe, Shrimp, Sole, Trout, Whiting, Yellowfish

3. Highly Beneficial Diary for Blood Type AB:

Cottage cheese, Farmer cheese, Feta, Goat cheese, Goat milk, Kefir, Mozzarella, Ricotta, Sour Cream, Yogurt

Avoid Dairy for Blood Type AB:

American, cheese, Blue cheese, Brie, Butter, Buttermilk, Camembert, Half & Half, Ice Cream, (pasteurized) Cow's milk, Parmesan, Provolone, Sherbet

4. Highly Beneficial Oils & Fats for Blood Type AB:

Olive oil, Walnut oil

Avoid Oils & Fats for Blood Type AB:

Cottonseed, Safflower, Sesame, Sunflower

5. Highly Beneficial Nuts for Blood Type AB:

Chestnuts, Peanuts, Peanut Butter, Walnut (Black/English)

Avoid Nuts for Blood Type AB:

Filbert, Poppy, Pumpkin, Sesame, Sunflower

6. Highly Beneficial Beans & Legumes for Blood Type AB:

Lentils, Green, Navy, Pinto, Soybean, Soy Tofu

Avoid Beans & Legumes for Blood Type AB:

Adzuki, Black bean, Black-Eyed peas, Fava, Garbanzo (chickpea), Kidney beans, Lima beans, Mung beans

7. Highly Beneficial Breads for Blood Type AB:

Brown Rice bread, Essene, Ezekiel, Rice cake, Rye, Soyflour,

Avoid Breads for Blood Type AB:
Corn bread, Corn muffins

8. Highly Beneficial Grains for Blood Type AB:
Amaranth, Millet, Oat Bran, Oatmeal, Rice, Rice flour, Rye flour, Spelt
Avoid Grains for Blood Type AB:
Buckwheat, Corn, Kasha, Grits, Kamut, Tapioca, Teff, Soba Noodles

9. Highly Beneficial Vegetables for Blood Type AB:
Alfalfa, Beet greens, Beets, Boccoli, Cauliflower, Celery, Collard greens, Cucumber, Dandelion, Eggplant, Garlic, Kale, Mushrooms, Parsley, Parsnip, Sweet potato, Yam
Avoid Vegetables for Blood Type AB:
Aloe, Artichoke, Caper, Corn, Shiitake mushroom, Black olive, Peppers (all), Pickles, Radish, Rhubarb

10. Highly Beneficial Fruits for Blood Type AB:
Cherry, Cranberry, Fig, Gooseberry, Grape, Grapefruit, Kiwi, Lemon, Pineapple, Plum, Watermelon
Avoid Fruits for Blood Type AB:
Avocado, Banana, Coconut, Guava, Mango, Melon, Orange, Persimmon, Pomegranate, Prickly pear, Quince, Sago Palm, Starfruit (carambola)

11. Highly Beneficial Juices for Blood Type AB:
Cabbage, Carrot, Celery, Cherry, Cranberry, Lemon
Avoid Juices for Blood Type AB:
Guava, Mango, Orange

12. Highly Beneficial Spices for Blood Type AB:

Curry, Garlic, Ginger, Horseradish, Blackstrap molasses, Oregano, Parsley

Avoid Spices for Blood Type AB:

Acacia, Allspice, Almond, Aspartame, Barley malt, Carrageenan, Cornstarch, Dextrose, Fructose, Gelatin, Guar gum, Invert sugar, Maltodextrin, MSG, Pepper, Sucanat, Tapioca, Vinegar, Brewer's yeast

13. Highly Beneficial Beverages for Blood Type AB:

Alfalfa, Astragalus, Burdock, Chamomile, Green tea, Fenugreek, Ginger, Ginseng, Hawthorn, Licorice root, Milk Thistle, Rose Hips, Strawberry leaf

Avoid Beverages for Blood Type AB:

Cayenne, Cornsilk, Coltsfoot, Hops, Red Clover, Rhubarb, Shepherd's Purse, Skullcap, Coffee, distilled Liquor, Soda, Black tea

Worth Repeating:

- *The key action here is to at least eliminate all or most of the major Avoid Foods listed in the previously advised **Short Version**, as they are the most damaging for Blood Type AB.*

Testimonials...

Dr. Peter D'Adamo (1996). *Eat Right 4 Your Blood Type.*

Case History: Chronic Fatigue Syndrome
Karen, 44 / Blood Type B

A patient named Karen suffered from Chronic Fatigue Syndrome her entire life. Her severe exhaustion prevented her from even holding a job. She endured debilitating headaches as well as back, neck and shoulder pain. Karen was a Blood Type B. After all other attempts at healing had failed, Karen was put on *a Blood Type B Diet. To her astonishment, within one week, Karen's symptoms had greatly lessened and she had a huge increase in energy. Most of her symptoms were resolved within a few weeks thereafter.*

Karen wrote a letter of thanks as follows:

"I have a whole new life! All my symptoms are practically gone and I hold two jobs having great energy 14 hours a day consistently. I believe diet is the key to this tremendous change. I am extremely active and feel like nothing can stop me. Thank you so very much!"

Case History: AutoImmune Disorder
Joan, 55 / Blood Type O

Joan suffered from chronic fatigue syndrome/Epstein Barr and arthritis. Joan's digestive system was so disrupted that she had severe gas, bloating and diarrhea from almost everything she ate. She was very weak and in chronic pain. She was *erroneously advised to eliminate red meat from her diet and add grains…the exact opposite of what a Blood Type O needs to thrive.*

After being put on a Blood Type O Diet which eliminated most grains and added red meat, Joan showed significant improvement in 2 weeks. Within 6 months, she advised she felt normal again. Joan confirmed that her renewed health and vitality endured as long as she adhered to her Blood Type O diet.

Case History: Lupus
Marcia, 30 / Blood Type A

178

Marcia was carried into her Doctor's office directly from the hospital Intensive care Unit where she had suffered kidney failure. She had been on shunt dialysis for several weeks and was scheduled for a kidney transplant within the next 6 months. Her diet history revealed that *she was eating a diet very high in dairy, wheat and red meat; the exact opposite foods that her Type A Blood needed to thrive.*

Marcia was put on a Blood Type A vegetarian diet along with some homeopathic preparations. Marcia's condition improved in only 2 weeks. Within 2 months, she was taken off dialysis and her kidney transplant surgery was canceled. Three years later, she still reported good health.

Case History: Anemia
Carol, 35 / Blood Type O

Carol was severely anemic. No matter what method was used to increase Carol's iron level, it invariably plummeted. After conferring with Dr. D'Adamo, Carol was put on a Blood Type O diet. This diet eliminated destructive food lectins which may have damaged Carol's red blood cells and obstructed the assimilation of iron in her body. After adhering to a high animal protein, low grain diet, Carol's iron levels began to rise up to normal.

It was determined that the incompatible "Avoid Foods" she was eating had agglutinated her intestinal tract preventing the assimilation of iron in her body.

Case History: Heart Disease
Wilma, 52 / Blood Type O

Wilma had advanced cardiovascular disease. She recently was released from the hospital where it was determined she had a cholesterol level of 350 (should be around 200 or less) and she had 80% blockage in three of her coronary arteries.

Type O's usually have a lower than average instance of heart disease. However, Wilma was eating a *diet high in processed oils and grains.* Wheat consumption in Type O's tends to create insulin sensitivity which causes the body to store fat and causes the triglycerides to become elevated. Dr. D'Adamo suggested *she eat more lean red meats in her diet and eliminate the processed oils and the grains.* But when she told this to her cardiologist, he was appalled and insisted on just putting her on cholesterol medication instead. Finally, Wilma agreed to try the Blood type O high meat diet and started walking for exercise.

After 6 months, Wilma reported having great energy. Despite eating ample amounts of red meat, her cholesterol dropped to 187…almost half of her original level. This is a classic example of the proven paradox that eating more red meat can actually drop the cholesterol levels of a Blood Type O.

Case History: Dangerously High Cholesterol
John, 23 / Blood Type O

John had alarmingly high cholesterol levels, high triglycerides and high blood sugar. It was especially frightening that he suffered these disorders at the very young age of 23 years old. Cardiology testing resulted in John being *advised that not even Cholesterol reducing drugs could help him.* In other words, John was destined to soon develop coronary heart disease and have a short life as a result of all these disorders. He also frequently suffered from sore throats and swollen glands.

The culprit was his diet. John was misadvised to follow a vegetarian diet which is the worst diet for a Blood Type O.

Once he switched to a Blood Type O diet, high in protein and red meats, amazingly he felt better in a few weeks. Within only 5 months, John's cholesterol, triglycerides and blood sugar levels all dropped into the normal range. Subsequent blood tests confirmed his levels remained stable while on the Blood Type O, high protein, high red meat diet.

Case History: Ear Infections
Tony, 7 / Blood Type B

Young Tony's mother advised her son was suffering from chronic ear infections, almost 15 per every winter season. He was on the escalating treadmill of being prescribed more and stronger antibiotics each time the infection recurred to no avail.

Upon questioning Tony about his diet he confirmed he eats "lots of chicken and corn"... 2 of the worst foods for a blood type B. Tony was put on a Blood Type B diet, eliminating all chicken, corn, peanuts and wheat. He went on to improve greatly, now having only one ear infection per year.

Case History: Crohn's Disease
Sarah, 35 / Blood Type B

Sarah had a severe case of Crohn's disease. After having undergone several surgeries on her bowels, she was anemic and suffered from chronic diarrhea.

Patient was put on the Blood Type B diet, which eliminates all chicken, corn, peanuts and wheat. Within 4 months, most of her digestive disorders including the chronic diarrhea completely disappeared.

Subsequently Sarah had surgery to remove some old scar tissue from a previous condition. Her surgeon advised *that he found no sign at all of active Crohn's disease in her abdominal cavity.*

Case History: Chronic Stomach Ulcers
Peter, 34 / Blood Type O

This Patient had suffered from chronic stomach ulcers since he was a child. He advised *that wheat was always a major part of his diet. Patient was put on a high protein Blood Type O diet, instructing that he strictly eliminate all wheat (corn and kidney beans).*

He was also advised to take Bladderwrack kelp and bismuth supplements. *In 6 weeks, Patient went to his gastroenterologist to have his stomach scoped. His doctor observed that 60% of his stomach lining had healed and appeared normal!*

A year later, Peter's condition was again assessed. His Doctor confirmed that his stomach ulcers were completely resolved.

Case History: Irritable Bowel Syndrome
Virginia, 26 / Blood Type O

Patient had severe irritable bowel syndrome which caused her to suffer alternately with severe constipation and then explosive diarrhea. She had chronic fatigue and was anemic. *Patient advised she adheres to a strict "Vegan/Vegetarian" diet. This is the worst possible diet for a Blood type O, and most often is severely problematic.*

Patient was instructed to switch to the Blood Type O diet as she was clearly unable to digest all the grains she was eating. She was put on a high protein diet of lean red meats, fish poultry and fresh fruits and vegetables which were all compatible with her blood type.

In 8 weeks, the patient appeared strong and robust, advising that her bowel problems were 90% better and she was enjoying normal energy again. A blood test confirmed that her anemia was gone. At 12 weeks, she was assessed as being free from all bowel problems and no longer needed a doctor's care.

Case History: Liver Deterioration
Sandra, 70 / Blood Type A

Sandra was suffering from a failing liver. She also had elevated liver enzymes and *ascites*, a condition where fluid builds up in the abdomen. This is a common effect of *advanced liver failure*. She was being treated with diuretics which was depleting her potassium, causing overwhelming fatigue. Sandra was very anemic, having a hematocrit (red blood cell count) of 27 with normal levels for a woman being 38.

Sandra was put on the Blood Type A vegetarian diet with some botanicals for liver support. *Within 4 months, all fluid retention in the abdomen disappeared and her liver enzymes dropped back to normal. Healthy red blood cells increased in number week by week. A year later, her red blood count had risen to 40.8.*

Case History: Severe Psoriasis
Marie, 66: Blood Type O

Marie was a difficult case. She had psoriasis lesions over 70% of her body. She also suffered from shortness of breath, difficulty walking and burning pain in her muscles and joints. Marie's medical records showed a 40 year history of sickness and surgeries. *Patient revealed that her typical diet was high in corn, wheat, nuts, processed foods along with high sugar and processed fats, all of which are a veritable curse for a Blood Type O.*

Marie was put on a Blood Type O diet along with vitamins and minerals. *Within 2 months, the swelling in her joints decreased markedly. She had improved breathing and the psoriasis lesions on her body were healing. She continued to improve each month.*

After 4 months, Marie's psoriasis was no longer evident. She had only slight swelling in her joints and her breathing was now normal.

Case History: Menstrual Problems
Patty, 45 / Blood Type O

Patty suffered from severe PMS, heavy menstrual bleeding, arthritis and high blood pressure. *She had been following a vegetarian diet,* so she was also anemic. Patty was put on a high protein, red meat, low grain Blood Type O diet.

Within only 2 months, Patty had an amazing turnaround in her health. Her arthritis was cured; Hypertension under control; PMS symptoms gone; Menstrual flow was normal.

This is yet another confirmation that a Blood Type O thrives on red meat, and is in fact inclined to contract multiple disorders in the absence of it in their diet.

Personal Testimonial…
Age 25: Joint pain in hips

Once upon a time, I was 25 and didn't know what I know now. I was a lover of popcorn. Back then when I didn't know any better, I used to eat that bad fat microwave popcorn. One night I ate 2 bags of it, all by myself. The next morning, I couldn't get out of bed because of the severe pain in my hips. Understand now, I was only 25 years old. So yes, I was more than a little alarmed that suddenly I could barely walk. I called my holistic Chiropractor, Dr. Lauria, who agreed to see me right away.

Dr. Lauria knew I was usually a very healthy, energetic person. When I lamented to him about my aching hips, he asked me one question, "*Did you eat corn last night*?"

I was astonished that he could know what the heck I ate the night before. He advised me way back then, that "*corn was bad for the joints*" for most blood types. I had no idea what blood type I was back then, but I made a quick and sure decision not to eat corn anymore. He further instructed me to *eat blueberries to rid my hips of the joint pain*. I proceeded to eat a pint of blueberries each day for 4 days. The pain was all gone by day 3. I just happen to love blueberries.

A decade later, I learned two very important facts: I was a Blood Type O; and yes, *Corn was detrimental to the joints of a Blood Type O.*

To this day, only once in a great while when I go to the movies I will have some popcorn, without *"butter"* of course. Because well, you know they don't use real butter right? (Movie popcorn "butter" is actually partially hydrogenated soybean oil (trans-fat), Flavacol/yellow dye, and Butylhydroquinone, a synthetic preservative.

…But, I'm sure you already knew this…;)

Knee Surgery Canceled…
Annie, 45 / Blood Type O

About 7 years ago, my dear friend Annie advised she had been having chronic knee pain and difficulty walking. She was scheduled to have knee surgery in a month. I asked her what Blood Type she was. Annie advised that she was a Blood Type O. Remembering my previous experience with corn overdose, I asked her "by any chance, *are you eating a lot of corn?*" My friend replied that *she eats corn 2 to 3 times a day! I advised her that corn is one of the worst foods for the joints of a Blood Type O.* I asked her to eliminate it completely from her diet along with bacon and kidney beans.

In about 2 weeks, Annie was a brand new person. She was walking fine and going up and down the stairs with ease. All of her joint pain was gone within a month. She canceled her knee surgery. Never needed it again, to this day.

Severe Arthritic Pain Relieved...
Harry, 60 / Blood Type O

Harry had chronic joint pain for years but he was referred to me because the pain in his hands had become so severe. Since this was a joint issue, I asked Harry what his blood type was. He advised he was a Blood Type O. I then asked him, *"Are you eating Pork, Kidney Beans and Corn, by any chance?"* He laughed and replied,*"Yes, and I had ALL THREE of those foods today!"* (Well, mystery solved.)

I asked him to eliminate all Pork, Ham and Bacon, Kidney beans and Corn from his diet. I suggested replacing the Pork with Red meat or Lamb, Chicken, Turkey, Halibut, Codfish or Red Snapper. I asked him to replace the Kidney beans with Back-Eyed peas, or black beans and replace all corn with Quinoa, Sweet Potatoes or rice. In only 1 week, the pain in Howard's hands diminished greatly. In 4 weeks, he felt overall relief from most of the joint pain he had suffered for many years.

Severe Digestive Disorders, Bloating
Tina, 45 / Blood Type O

Tina was suffering from acute stomach bloating, indigestion and severe constipation. She also had gained 40 pounds, had low energy and was feeling depressed. She advised her diet included a bagel first thing in the morning (wheat flour) and sodas throughout the day. Tina advised she was a Blood Type O.

I automatically asked her to eliminate the top worst *Avoid Foods* for an O: No Corn, Kidney beans, Navy beans, Lentils, Pork, or Wheat/Wheat flour. Soda's should be eliminated no matter what your blood type is, as they are destructive to the teeth and to the arteries. I also advised that bagels are often very constipating. Eating one every day just multiplies the problem.

Since her intestinal tract was so impacted, Tina went on a three day cleanse of raw fruits and vegetable smoothies with Chia Seeds and raw Coconut Oil. Thereafter, she strictly adhered to a high protein, low grain Blood Type O Diet. I asked that she switch out the bagels for Oatmeal and eggs in the morning and that she add raw unrefined Coconut Oil to every meal, as it cleans out parasites and leans down the body as well. Lastly, I asked her *to replace all grains and carbs with the following*: Sweet potatoes, Quinoa, Oatmeal, Rye, Brown rice, Ezekiel bread, Bananas and Apples. These carbs are *Beneficial or Neutral for Blood Type O.*

After only 1 week of no sodas and following a Blood Type O Diet, her stomach was getting flatter and much less distended with gasses. After only 2 weeks, she felt much better overall and had lost 15 pounds (remember she did a liquid cleanse for 3 days*.) As the weeks went by, her health markedly improved in all areas. She had regular elimination, no bloating, renewed energy. Her mental state of wellbeing was greatly elevated. She advised feeling "like a new person."*

187

By now, I hope you are both amazed and convinced that simple dietary adjustments have been proven to bring stunning and life-changing healing.

NEXT ACTION:
"Follow the Recipe,"
   ...1,2,3...

1). Learn your Blood type
   with an at home blood typing kit, Amazon.

2). Plug the Holes in Your Boat...
   LISTEN TO YOUR BLOOD TYPE!
ELIMINATE all or most of the "Major Avoid"/"Dirty Dozen" foods for your blood type, which are listed in the **Short Version** at the beginning of each Blood Type section.

3). ADD many of the "Major Beneficial Foods"
   listed at the beginning of your Blood Type section.

   Enjoy your increased energy, weight loss and better health!

Small changes can cause extraordinary results in your Health and in Your Life.

Please pause here to lead others to better health, by leaving a Book Review now on Amazon.

Using just 1 minute of your time, it is in your power to change someone's health and someone's life, for the better…

Chapter Four

3,000 YEAR OLD SECRET
"Oil Pulling"

I believe this chapter will just fascinate you! Because Oil Pulling is the easiest and oldest secret for body detoxing ever discovered. Yet, I have never met anyone who wasn't initially skeptical about the effectiveness of this incredibly simple practice which enables the body to heal itself in the most amazing way.

Oil Pulling began in Ayurvedic medicine, an ancient and proven system of healing and preventative care that began in India approximately 3,000 years ago. In 1971, the Indian government founded the Indian Medical Council to establish the standard of quality of Indian Medicine for undergraduate and postgraduate education. Both then and now, Ayurvedic medicine is one of the most highly esteemed, empirical sources of healing protocols in existence. Ayurvedic practices are still widely used today either alone or along with modern medicine. In alignment with most Ayurvedic modalities, *Oil Pulling brings both a curative and preventive aspect to the body, in the easiest possible way.*

The invaluable information in this chapter is derived in part from the exhaustive research results of Roberta M. Meehan, Ph.D.; Dr. F. Karach, M.D.; Weston A. Price, D.D.S.; Dr. Bruce Fife, C.N., N.D., and many others. The following testimonials are extrapolated from Dr. Fife's book

Oil Pulling Therapy (2008). It was the following amazing transformations that spurred me to include Oil Pulling into my personal daily health routine:

Chronic Fatigue, Fibromyalgia, Depression
Theresa / Melbourne, Australia

Theresa had been suffering from Chronic Fatigue for 14 years. She was confined to bed and had limited mobility. Her Fibromyalgia condition caused her to be in chronic pain. She had no quality of life. Even worse, she was depressed and at times suicidal.

Theresa started Oil Pulling for 20 minutes every day and advised she saw improvements in her body, day by day. *After only a few weeks of Oil Pulling, she attests she has prevailed over 2 "incurable" chronic disorders. She confirms she is now "fit and active", declaring, "Oil Pulling has given me my life back!"*

Arthritis and Skin Disorders
Carolina / Puerto Vallarta, Mexico

Although Carolina was a young girl, she was enduring painful arthritic symptoms in her shoulders, hips, feet, knees and neck. She began Oil Pulling for 20 minutes each day. Each week brought more improvement to her symptoms. After only 2 months, she reported that all her aches were gone and had not returned as of this point, 9 months later. Also, her chronic skin condition called keratosis pilaris had disappeared. She went on to confirm that her gums and tongue were pinker, her teeth were whiter and the dark circles under her eyes had lightened. Lastly, she advised that her sleep is better, her energy increased, and that she feels much better overall.

Carolina advised *she will never stop Oil Pulling and recommends that you should try it for 30 days to see good results.*

Loose Teeth Tightened, Overall Revitalization
Louis / West Bountiful, Utah

Louis was quite clear about how deeply impressed he and his wife were with their Oil Pulling results. He advised that after only 1 month of Oil Pulling, he knew it was *"the most powerful therapy he ever discovered."* Louis confirmed that he and his wife are now sleeping much better, have greatly improved digestion and their muscle aches and pains had disappeared. Even his loose teeth had tightened up. Lastly, at 65 years old, he now feels he has a younger body overall. But my favorite part of his testimonial was this ultimate declaration:

"Anyone who doesn't try this for a month is dumber than a rock."

*(I admit, it was this last statement
that spurred me to try Oil Pulling ;)*

What the Heck is Oil Pulling...?

Oil Pulling is a daily practice that powerfully detoxifies the body, enabling it to efficiently heal itself. It originated in ancient Ayurvedic Medicine. Although the technique is very simple, it renders very impressive results. Because of its simplicity, many people dismiss Oil Pulling as too good to be true; but in fact, it is based upon a long-standing scientific fact that *almost all sickness and disease begin in the mouth.* Hundreds of scientific studies have confirmed the very important fact that *the mouth is the door to the body's health.* A mountain of Medical and Dental research journals have reconfirmed this *direct link between oral health and systemic disease.*

Oil Pulling is performed by simply taking 1-2 teaspoons of an edible oil into the mouth and swishing it around (like mouthwash) for 20 minutes. Then spit it out. That's it.

So this is the part where you say, "you're kidding right?"

Now open your mind to receive the scientific results and hard evidence that validate this simple yet powerful detoxing therapy.

Simple Science says...

The human mouth harbors approximately 600 kinds of viruses, bacteria, fungi and parasites. At any given time, there are about 10 BILLION microbes (germs) in your mouth and saliva. *How disturbing is that?* Most viruses and bacteria have *fatty cell walls; and fat attracts fat.* So the action of simply "swishing" an edible oil back and forth through the teeth causes the oil you put in your mouth to *"attract and trap"* a multitude of those oral microbes. Like a powerful magnet, Oil Pulling attracts the microbes in your mouth and holds onto them until you literally spit them out. The oil you put into your mouth is initially clear, but when you spit it out, it is thick and cloudy, because after 20 minutes of swishing, the oil is just loaded with germs and toxins it has removed from your mouth. *Both simple and wonderful.*

Any edible oil would work: Coconut Oil, Olive Oil, Avocado Oil, Sesame oil, etc. Since you are NOT swallowing this oil, the type of oil you use is really irrelevant. I Oil Pull for 20 minutes every day using unrefined Coconut Oil, because I simply believe it to be the best of all oils. The fact remains *that any edible oil is a fat* which attracts the fatty cell walls of the microbes in your mouth. To reiterate, *the oil does not kill the microbes; it attracts and traps them (okay like a mousetrap) until you physically spit them out down the drain.*

Now, doing this only once will not have a huge impact on your health; but all studies confirm that *doing it faithfully for 20 minutes each day will <u>deeply detox your body</u>, relieve your overworked immune system and substantially improve systemic health disorders which are decades old.*

- ***Almost Every Disease begins in the Mouth.***

Says Who...?

In 1923, Dr. Weston A. Price and a *team of 60 leading scientists* performed an *exhaustive 25-year study* confirming that (with few exceptions) *"all disease begins in the mouth."* Dr. Price et al performed hundreds of experiments confirming this fact. His discoveries were well documented in a multi-volume publication consisting of 1,174 pages. Later, his findings were reconfirmed by a team of researchers along with Charles Mayo, M.D., founder of the world-famous Mayo Clinic, *whose 20-year study further proved that the mouth is the focal point of infections and disease in the body.* The lead scientist, *Dr. Edward C. Rosenow, recorded over 200 scientific reports on this fact, reconfirming Dr. Price's conclusions which were both amazing and alarming, as follows:*

- *Bacteria from the mouth of patients with specific health disorders created the same disorders when injected into laboratory animals.*

For example, bacteria from the mouth of a patient with a liver infection caused liver infection when injected into a lab animal. Bacteria taken from the mouth of an arthritis patients

194

caused arthritis when injected into lab animals. *These astonishing findings exactly matched the previous findings of Dr. Price proving that oral bacteria was the root cause of the vast majority of systemic diseases.*

How Oil Pulling Enables Your Body to Heal itself…

The sum total of all the microbes in your body is known as your *toxic load.* Over months, years and decades, this *toxic load* level grows so extremely high that your immune system becomes overwhelmed. Your overworked immune system is so busy fighting your *high toxic load* that it has little or no remaining capacity to fight anything else. The result of this is that infections, disorders and disease prevail.

Oil Pulling "pulls" (attracts and traps) disease-causing bacteria and toxins from your mouth, gums, from under the tongue and from between your teeth, allowing you to literally spit them out. The *cumulative effect* of Oil Pulling is that, day by day, you are removing more and more microbes, reducing the massive overabundance from your mouth and body, thereby *lowering your toxic load.* In a relatively short time, *practicing* **Oil Pulling greatly relieves your overwhelmed immune system from this toxic burden, enabling it to heal your body of many disorders that may have existed for years**.

The Short Version:

- **The practice of Oil Pulling powerfully "frees up" your immune system so it can protect and heal your body, as it was designed to do.**

"Why Do I Care if My Gums Bleed …?"

Your mouth is a *microbial swimming pool,* brimming with viruses, bacteria, fungi and parasites. These germs can remain relatively harmless, unless and until they find a way into the bloodstream. Bleeding gums or any break in the gum, like a cut, puncture or ulcer, allow these vipers to enter the bloodstream and wreak systemic disorder and disease in a multitude of ways. The mouth is very capillary dense, especially your gums and under your tongue. The tissue of the gums is packed with tiny blood vessels. *When gums become inflamed (e.g., bleeding gums) they become highly permeable, meaning microbes can easily pass into them. Ignoring your bleeding gums allows a multitude of germs to pass easily through your unhealthy gums and into your bloodstream…without you knowing a thing.*

Periodontitis / Gum Disease…

Gum disease (periodontitis) is like having the equivalent of a 9 square inch open wound. That is approximately the amount of permeable tissue in your mouth that is vulnerable to receiving microbes passing through it every day. Once these germs enter the bloodstream, they can target any organ or area of the body. It is well documented that oral germs entering the bloodstream have caused arthritis, heart disorders (endocarditis), diabetes and other systemic diseases. That is why a Dentist gives antibiotics to a patient before performing a procedure that will cut or puncture the gums. Gum disease begins with swollen, bleeding gums (gingivitis). It progresses gradually so that you may not notice it or think it is important.

Early symptoms of gum disease are swollen or bleeding gums, pockets forming between teeth and the gum line, loose teeth, chronic bad breath, and sometimes a metallic taste in the mouth. With advanced gum disease, gums shrink away from the loose teeth creating gaps where toxins and bacteria grow below the gumline. Over time, these bacteria destroy the connective tissue and bone in the infected area. Even worse, at this point these toxins have spread into the bloodstream where they wreak havoc in other areas of the body.

This is why it is so important to catch gum disease at the *early stage*, when you notice your gums are bleeding. At this point, it is highly likely that these symptoms are *reversible.*

- *People with gum disease are 3x more likely to have a heart attack than those with healthy gums.*

The Farmers Knew All Along ...

For centuries, Farmers were well aware of the relationship between poor oral health and disease. Before they purchased livestock, they would check the gums and teeth, because the Farmers *knew if the animal had poor oral health, then it was highly probable that the animal was unhealthy...or soon would be.*

Who Else Knew this Besides the Farmers...?

So says Robert J. Genco, D.D.S., Ph.D. from the University of Buffalo who conducted a 10-year study with over 1,300 people. *His results confirmed that heart disease developed 3x more in those participants who had gum disease.* The National Health and Nutritional Examination Study *concur that people with inflammation of the gums have at least a 25% greater risk of heart disease.*

This is why Oil Pulling is an invaluable remedy and an incredibly simple way to save your gums, your teeth and your overall health.

Upon hearing about Oil Pulling, Dr. Bruce Fife freely admits he was very skeptical at first, as the reported results of healing seemed almost miraculous. But the surprising amount of research done on Oil Pulling and the sheer volume of success stories drove him to perform his own experiment. He began oil pulling for 20 minutes 3x a day, to speed up expected results. Dr. Fife was shocked to see that the *results for him were immediate*. His sinuses started draining heavily, he developed temporary hoarseness in his throat, he had brief headaches and was coughing up mucus. Although his body was imitating sickness, he did not feel sick. He realized this sudden release of toxins from his body was evidence that he was going through a *healing crisis,* which means his body was quickly ridding itself of stored up toxins.

In his Book, *Oil Pulling Therapy*, Dr. Fife affirms he was amazed to see the following results:

For 30 years, he had suffered from painful dermatitis on his face and chest. His skin would flare up turning very red, becoming itchy, painful and even peeling. The worst flare ups would cause his skin to actually crack and ooze. Over the years, his skin problem worsened causing his face and chest to be inflamed almost every day. After choosing to improve his diet, his skin condition improved but still persisted.

The very first day Dr. Fife started Oil Pulling, the redness in his face disappeared and he had no subsequent flare ups. Remarkably, even his lifelong battle with severe (he called it "massive") dandruff was finally won. Dandruff is a fungus that lives in the skin. Yet after only 3 weeks of Oil Pulling, his lifelong dandruff had cleared up by 95%.

Additionally, a wart he had on his face for 20 years, disappeared. Warts are caused by a virus. Dr. Fife came to the stunning conclusion that this simple act of Oil Pulling was seemingly "sucking out" the bacteria, fungi and viruses from his body, *lowering its toxic load.*

Dr. Fife is an Author, a Nutritionist and a Naturopathic physician who affirms that *"Oil Pulling is one of the most powerful detox and healing therapies I have ever encountered."* (Fife, 2008)

Chronic Blood Disorder & Arthritis Cured...

Much of the credit for reintroducing this ancient oil swishing practice is given to Dr. F. Karach, M.D. who attests having remarkable results with his patients using this method, which he called *"Oil Pulling."* In a presentation held in the Ukraine which was given to a global audience of medical practitioners, Dr. Karach revealed his amazing rediscovery of how powerful Oil Pulling was for healing or greatly relieving many disorders and diseases. He affirmed that the action of pushing and pulling oil through the teeth (for at least 20 minutes) *literally pulls toxins and germs out of the body, allowing the body to heal itself.* He advised that this method works on headaches, bronchitis, toothache, eczema, ulcers, intestinal disorders, insomnia and disorders of the blood, nerves and stomach.

Dr. Karach revealed that for 15 years he had endured a chronic blood disease which was healed by Oil Pulling. He further claimed that his crippling case of chronic *arthritis was also cured within one week of Oil Pulling.* He advised that sunflower oil can be used but went on to say that any oil should work. Dr. Karach confirms that *by relieving stress from the immune system, the body is then enabled to heal itself so that chronic and acute illnesses are cured or relieved (Karach, 1992).*

Dr. Karach's presentation was recorded in a Medical Journal in Calcutta, India in 1992.

After learning of Dr. Karach's work, a retired military officer named Tummala Koteswara Rao began Oil Pulling with his wife in January 1993. He recorded the following successful results:

At 63 years old, *Mr. Rao attests that Oil Pulling has cured him of 40 years of asthma, sleeplessness, heart palpitations and digestive problems.* He further claims that his wife, 56 years old, was cured of 30 years of migraine headaches, and 40 years of varicose veins, ulcers, arthritis and high blood pressure. Mr. Rao was so impressed with these incredible results that he wrote pamphlets on the subject. He even published newspaper articles about it in the Telugu Daily for three years. Mr. Rao went on to give 1,000 lectures on Oil Pulling in the following 12 years. During this time, he had received approximately 1,200 letters from people rejoicing in their success. Mr. Rao affirms that *"all of these people attested they were cured"* from their disorders from Oil Pulling, after traditional medical treatments had been repeatedly ineffective. (Rao, 1996)

(…and you thought it was just all woo-woo, didn't you…?)

- *Fun Fact:*
  Oil Pulling has also been shown to whiten teeth.

What is the "Germiest" Part of the Body…?
Surprise…It's your Mouth.

Dr. Roberta M. Meehan, Ph.D. advised she used to perform a very odd and very fun experiment in her microbiology classroom each semester. She would have her students take saliva samples from the mouth of a dog and from a newborn baby's mouth, by swabbing. The results were consistent. Each time, it was proven that the *dog's mouth was relatively free of bacteria, whereas the newborn baby's mouth was full of bacteria.* This revelation shocked her students every time. It shocked me too, frankly. This is the premise upon which is built the adage *"all disease begins in the mouth."*

Hundreds of species of fungi, viruses and protozoa along with 600 kinds of bacteria live quietly in your mouth. Even *Streptococcus mutans* bacteria live there. They feed on sugars and refined carbohydrates and are the main cause of cavities in your teeth. As this bacteria digest the sugars in your mouth, they release an *acidic waste produc*t. Over time, the enamel of your teeth is then eroded by this acid by-product. Unfortunately, brushing your teeth has little effect on these bacteria that have set up shop in your mouth.

Did You Know...

- *In days of old, Dentists would pull an infected tooth to cure systemic disease.*

- *The bottom of your shoe has less bacteria than your mouth.*

- *There are less bacteria per square inch of your toilet seat then in your mouth.*
    (...how do you like me now...?)

Toxic Pumps in Your Mouth...

In the wake of extensive research, a vast amount of scientific evidence has been published confirming that gum disease, tooth decay, amalgam (silver) fillings and root canals are major contributors to overall ill health (*Chapter 6, Oral Health*). Hippocrates, the "Father of Modern Medicine," declared 2,700 years ago that *pulling an infected tooth often cured the patient of a systemic disorder,* especially arthritis. This protocol became so successful that it was regularly practiced by Dentists all the way up to the early 1900's.

However, with the introduction of antibiotics, the impact of oral infections on the body was no longer a primary concern. Dentists quickly adopted the practice of prescribing antibiotics to the patient instead of pulling the infected tooth. Please note, this is not to say that every tooth infection means the tooth should be pulled. But when a patient's tooth is badly infected, where the infection has spread into the root, and that infection flares up each time the antibiotics run out, then there is a much deeper problem there. Severe and chronic tooth infection is a *toxic pump,* which silently and steadily leaks toxins and bacteria into your bloodstream. I explain this in great detail in Chapter 6. Meanwhile, *let's focus here on reversing the early symptoms of gum disease and saving your teeth.*

I taught Oil Pulling in my Health and Wellness classes for years. Without fail, each class had many of my students reporting with excitement that their *gums had stopped bleeding and their loose teeth became tighter after only 2-3 weeks of Oil Pulling.* I was a direct and delighted witness to these oral transformations which I will share in the Testimonials at the end of this chapter.

The KLES Institute Study...

A study was conducted in Belgaum, India, under the Department of Preventive and Community Dentistry at the KLES Institute of Sciences. The purpose of this study was to ascertain whether or not Oil Pulling had a curative result on patients with gingivitis and plaque.

All participants had mild to moderate gingivitis and plaque. After 45 days of Oil Pulling, it was determined that *plaque was reduced by 30% and gingivitis was reduced by over 52%*. The reduction in gingivitis was 7x greater than those just using antiseptic mouthwash. Lastly, it was also reconfirmed that Oil Pulling had no negative side effects whatsoever. These findings were recorded in scientific journals.

V.H.N.S.N. College Study, Virudhunagar, India...

The purpose of this study was to determine the effect of Oil Pulling on the amount of *Streptococcus mutans* in the mouth. These bacteria are the main contributors to tooth decay. Test subjects were asked to Oil Pull for 40 days. Their oral bacteria was measured both before and after study.

It was discovered that Oil Pulling had reduced Streptococcus mutans by 33% in 40 days. The study concluded that Oil Pulling "was effective in reducing bacterial growth and adhesion."

The Purpose of Saliva...

Saliva plays a strong part in keeping our mouths healthy. It contains a blend of antibodies, enzymes and nutrients that play a part in helping to protect the teeth and gums.

- *About 34 ounces of saliva is produced by your mouth each day.*

- *About 2.5 billion bacterial cells are in 1 teaspoon of saliva.*

This multitude of microbes live in different areas of your mouth, some preferring the gums or the back of the tongue, others preferring the teeth and the roof of the mouth. As you can see, it is almost impossible to efficiently clean all areas of the mouth by brushing your teeth. Mouthwash may temporarily give you that clean feeling, but it does not *attract and trap microbes and prepare them for disposal like Oil Pulling easily does.*

What Say the Surveys...?
The Andhra Jyoti Survey, 1996...

Founded in 1960, Andhra Jyoti is the third largest Telugu language daily newspaper in India. It is also the oldest one. In 1996, this newspaper proposed a survey to its readers for the purpose of collecting evidence on the effectiveness of Oil Pulling. There were over 1,000 participants.

The results of the survey showed that out of these 1,000 participants, 927 that is **89% reported having been cured of one or more diseases**. Only 11% advised they had no meaningful results. The recorded healings in descending order were as follows:

- Aches and pains throughout body
- Asthma, allergies and respiratory conditions
- Eczema, pigmentation and skin problems
- Digestive problems
- Constipation

- Joint pain and Arthritis
- Diabetes
- Hemorrhoids
- Polycystic kidney, neurofibroma and polio

The Pioneer Match Industries Survey, 2005...

Conducted in Tamil Nadu, India, the Pioneer Match Industries survey consisted of 144 females. At the end of 25 days of Oil Pulling, the participants were asked to rate the overall effectiveness it had on their health. Their report was as follows:

- 93% reported improvement.
- 56% = Good or Very Good Results
- 5% advised no benefit.

One participant in this study was diabetic and on medication. *She reported she was able to cut her diabetes medication dosage in half after only 20 days of Oil Pulling.* Being excited by these results, she continued Oil Pulling even when the survey had ended. After Oil Pulling for 40 days, she reported having much better energy and *was off all diabetes medication, yet her blood sugar level remained normal.*

- **As you can see by these many Oil Pulling studies, not every single participant had measurable results; but the vast majority reported dramatic results.**

Oil Pulling has also been shown to be highly effective in treating Oral Candida which is a fungus that usually appears as a white coating on the tongue or white patches

205

on the inner cheeks or on the roof of the mouth. Oral Candida can lead to an oral infection called thrush. Left untreated, oral Candida can spread throughout the body as a systemic yeast infection. *Systemic Candidiasis* adversely affects the blood brain, eyes, bones and major organs of the body. Some Candida usually exists in the body. It is normally harmless, unless the patient has a compromised immune system. Receiving chemotherapy, taking strong antibiotics or too many rounds of antibiotics can also trigger the overgrowth of Candida in the body. *The daily practice of Oil Pulling is the simplest most effective way to keep this fungus in check, preventing its overgrowth and averting the more serious problems that come with it.*

The Simplicity of Oil Pulling is also its Dichotomy...

Most people doubt the effectiveness of simply swishing oil in their mouth. Yet for thousands of years, this act of swishing oil in your mouth for 20 minutes a day has been proven highly effective in healing chronic disorders and improving overall health. Lastly, this very simple practice has no known negative side effects and does not interfere with any medication.

So, why in the world would you NOT try it ...?

Testimonials...

A huge thank you to my Aunt Mary who introduced me to Oil Pulling Therapy many years ago. Acquiring this single Seed of Wisdom enabled me to teach its power to hundreds of people, with much success.

The Power of One Seed Planted...

Edema, Severe Joint and Foot Pain healed
Mary, 75 Years Old

Mary was a wonderful bright spirited person trapped inside a malfunctioning body. When Mary joined my class in 2017, she had edema (fluid/swelling) in her legs with severe pain in her ankles and feet which greatly impaired her walking. She dreaded the idea of having to use a walker, or worse, that she may soon be needing a wheelchair to get around. *She advised that on a scale of 1 to 10, her pain was an 11.*

I asked Mary to start Oil Pulling every day for 20 minutes using Coconut Oil. Each week, she advised that she felt less and less pain, and saw a gradual reduction of swelling in her legs. *By the end of my 5-week class, she was 90% back to normal. After 6 weeks, Mary came into my next class to give her testimonial that she had almost no remaining edema or pain in her legs and feet. She further attested that she was now walking normally without help and that her pain level went from an 11…to a zero!*

Simple practice; Powerful results.

Stage 2 Gum Disease healed
Kristen, 32 Years Old

Kristen was a young, beautiful girl. But when she smiled her swollen inflamed gums were the first thing you saw. Her gums were so swollen that they protruded past her teeth. When she came to my class, Kristen advised she has had swollen and bleeding gums for many years. There were also deep pockets (gaps) between her teeth and her gums so that she could put her fingernail into them. It was not surprising to hear that she also had many loose teeth. I was afraid that this beautiful girl would lose her teeth by the time she was 40. I asked her to Oil Pull 20 minutes every day with Coconut Oil.

It took only 1 week for Kristen's gums to stop bleeding. After 2 weeks, she advised the open pockets over each tooth were closing up. After a month, Kristen confirmed to my class that her gums were back to normal pink, healthy, with no swelling, no bleeding, and her loose teeth had all tightened up! We all cheered for her victory! After 5 years of gum disease, it took only 4 weeks of Oil Pulling to heal her gums and save her teeth.

Edema & Severe Joint Pain Gone
Terry, 70 Years Old

Terry was a strong spirited 70-year-old. She had a law degree and was also a Homeopathic Doctor. Sadly, over the years she had developed edema (fluid buildup) in her legs as well as severe pain in her hips and legs. This resulted in her needing a wheelchair to get around. Terry joined my Wellness Class and learned about Oil Pulling. She decided to start Oil Pulling for 20 minutes every day with Coconut Oil. The first week, she advised she had a raspy throat, a great deal of mucus coming from her nose and "phantom headaches" that mysteriously came and went. She recognized that her body was going through a "healing crisis," that her body was dumping toxins at a rapid pace. *Each week, her symptoms lessened further. By the end of the 5 week class, Terry was having minimal joint pain and greatly reduced edema. By 6 weeks, she had abandoned her wheelchair completely.*

Yep. Oil Pulling.

Loose Teeth and Toenail Fungus Healed
Michelle, 50 Years Old

I observed that Michelle was a very fit 50-year-old when she joined my class in 2018. Her complaints were that she had loose teeth, which suggested a substantial amount of Gingivitis was present as in stage 2 gum disease. I asked her to Oil Pull every day for 20 minutes with Coconut Oil.

After only a few short weeks, Michelle advised that not only did her loose teeth tighten up, but a bad case of toenail fungus she had for many years just disappeared. It was a double win for Michelle.

Rhabdomyolysis, Rare Muscle Disease Healed
John, 45 Years Old
(Testimonial also in Chapter 1)

In 2017, a woman named Claudia came to my Health and Wellness Class. Claudia was distraught, advising that her husband, John, had a rare muscle disease called Rhabdomyolysis. This is a disease that causes muscle tissue breakdown and the release of a damaging protein into the blood which ultimately causes kidney damage. *The Doctors advised no hope of cure*, only giving her husband 5 prescriptions: a muscle relaxer, antidepressant, sleeping pill, blood pressure medicine and painkillers. As a result, this poor man's condition only worsened. He couldn't walk even short distances without being in severe pain and needing to be on oxygen. Finally, he ended up depressed and in a wheelchair at the young age of 45 years old. John also had been out of work and on Disability for the past three years. After much prayer and heartache, Claudia confessed she joined my class as a last-minute hope. She was desperate to find a resolution for her husband and for the hugely negative impact his poor health has had on their young family.

At this juncture, let me repeat the most beautiful thing about using raw Coconut Oil and/or Oil Pulling to treat a disorder: These 2 protocols have never been found to worsen any condition or otherwise cause harm. So, *even if you don't know the exact cause of an illness, eating Coconut Oil and practicing Oil Pulling each day will most likely improve symptoms and many times, will also eradicate the cause. This fact is a timeless Gem of Wisdom that you need to tuck inside your Wellness Treasure Chest, forever. Pursuant to this knowledge, I was undeterred by this man's "incurable" diagnosis.*

As was my creed, I delivered my usual unwavering instructions to John:
1) *THROW OUT ALL PROCESSED FATS AND OILS* from your kitchen.
2) Use ONLY unrefined Coconut Oil for cooking, for everything.
2) Eat 8 Tablespoons of unrefined Coconut Oil per day, every day.
4) Do *Oil Pulling* 20 minutes every day.
5) Take 5 drops of Cellfood in water 2x a day (*Chapter 10, Cellfood*).

I also instructed that John drink 2 raw fruit smoothies per day with raw Coconut Oil and with 20-30 gram protein (from protein powder) because muscles needed protein for regrowth and repair.

Each week in class Claudia reported that John was rigidly following my instructions as he was very desperate to regain his life. In THREE WEEKS, Claudia came into my classroom in tears, *revealing that her husband had just taken their 4 children to the Zoo where he walked around for 2 hours without needing oxygen, painkillers… or his wheelchair! He was also off his blood pressure medication and antidepressants. Claudia and her husband were elated…and, oh so was I.*

Claudia later confirmed that by week 6 John had abandoned his wheelchair completely and that he was off all 5 medications.

John's results were life-changing for him and for his family. He took back his health and his life in 6 weeks.

Simple choices; profound results.

Seasonal Allergies Gone, Growths Reduced, Whiter Teeth Paula, Utah

After a year of Oil Pulling for 20 minutes a day with organic Coconut Oil, Paula confirms her seasonal allergies have disappeared, her skin looks better and her teeth are whiter. Yellow spots on her teeth from Fluorosis (from too much fluoride) had lessened and the vertical grooves that had plagued her teeth since kindergarten are now gone. Growths on her cheeks that were 10 years old have decreased in size with one growth disappearing altogether.

She confirms she is enjoying overall better health from the practice of Oil Pulling.

Reduced Leg Cramps, Improved Energy
Henah, India

Henah asserts that after only one week of Oil Pulling, she has reduced leg cramps, improvement in her cracked heels and is also enjoying great energy.

Acne and Arthritis cleared up
June, Canada

After Oil Pulling twice a day for 5 weeks with unrefined Virgin Coconut Oil, June advises that for the first week she experienced a scratchy throat, a lot of mucus which she coughed up and that she was spitting out a substantial amount of phlegm. June was going through a *Healing Crisis* whereby the body acutely rids itself of toxins. When this phase ended, she started sleeping soundly.

June confirms the acne flare-ups she had suffered for 25 years were lessening to nothing. Her teeth were whiter, her gums pinker and she had reduced tartar on her bottom teeth. Lastly, the arthritis in her hands vanished where previously they were always stiff and painful.

June concludes by asserting that nothing has had such remarkable changes to her health as Oil Pulling has. She states, it "quite literally changed her life."

Sinus Infection Cleared Up
Mick, Alabama

Mick started Oil Pulling for 20 minutes a day as a possible remedy for his chronic sinus infections. He used Sunflower Oil. After a day or two his sinuses opened up and drained out and all the pressure he suffered was gone.

Mick advised that he sometimes had a "gag reflex" when he first started Oil Pulling, *but recommends that if you persist with this practice, you will be as amazed as he is.*

Chronic Sinus Infections and Bad Breath cleared up
Fina, Nigeria

Since childhood, Fina had endured chronic sinus infections with copious drainage of mucus on a daily basis. Bad breath came along with the package. After 6 months of Oil Pulling, Fuma confirms *"amazing results."* Her nasal *passages have been cleaned out, her sinuses are clear, and she now has a clean, healthy breath.*

Teeth Tighter, Healed Loose Skin inside Mouth

Tina, California

After only 8 days of Oil Pulling for 20 minutes a day, Tina advised her *"amazement"* at the results. Her gums had firmed up and her teeth were *whiter and tighter. She confirms she also had a flap of excess skin in her mouth which completely disappeared from the Oil Pulling. Tina claims that Oil Pulling "works for her and she's sticking to it!"*

Goiter / Thyroid Tumor Shrunk
Veronica, Canada

Ten years ago, Veronica developed a Goiter (thyroid tumor) that was sizable enough to be visible. No medication, diet change or supplement impacted its size. It had not grown any bigger but it had not grown any smaller in 10 years.

Veronica began Oil Pulling. She advised she had a metallic taste in her mouth the first day. Each day after Oil Pulling she would be spitting out mucus and phlegm. Then to her amazement her Goiter began shrinking. She attest that *it shrunk so much in size that she believed a doctor would not even be able to find it now. Lastly, she saw that her teeth were much whiter.*

Veronica loves the fact that Oil Pulling is so effective and so easy to do. She asserts she will be using Oil Pulling in her daily health routine for the rest of her life.

Chronic Lymph Node Infection Healed
"Convinced" from Canada

After only 3 days of Oil Pulling, "Convinced" confirms that his chronically infected lymph node has reduced to its normal size and is free of all swelling and infection.

During his first few days of Oil Pulling he had headaches (from his "Healing Crises"). After 2 weeks, he further attests that his teeth are whiter, his skin is smoother, and that he is sleeping much better.

Bursitis and Arthritis Cleared Up
Lauren, New Mexico

Lauren advised she had severe pain in her shoulder and arm because of Bursitis and Arthritis. The pain was bad during the day but severe at night. She heard about Oil Pulling and decided to try it. *After Oil Pulling with Coconut Oil, she attests she was almost pain free in just a few weeks.*

Severe Burn Out Reversed
Dan, New Jersey

Dan lamented that he was suffering from acute exhaustion. His symptoms were shooting pains all over his body and dizzy spells as well as pain in his back and abdomen. Seeking relief, he started Oil Pulling.

Dan asserts that his symptoms started reducing in severity the very first day he Oil Pulled. He confirms that after only 4 days of Oil Pulling, all his symptoms had disappeared completely. In concussion he states his healing "felt like a Miracle!"

Skin Rash and Gaps in Gums Cleared Up
Kelly, Australia

Kelly advised she had a gap that formed in her mouth between her dental bridge and her gums.

After only a week of Oil Pulling that gap just closed up. Her gum discoloration disappeared and the plaque on her teeth was gone. Kelly attests she also had sore and swollen gums which hurt when she ate, but that went away in the very first week of Oil Pulling. Also, after a few weeks of Oil Pulling, a skin rash she had for some time just cleared up. Lastly, she confirms that during her 6 months of Oil Pulling, she has not had any flu or sickness.

Kelly advised she did Oil Pulling each morning before breakfast, using Virgin Olive Oil. Then she rinses her mouth out with warm water. Her results were so successful, she had her children start doing it each day. She affirms their Dentist is amazed at how clean and free of plaque her children's teeth are. She advises that people should persist through the *"healing crises"* that may occur in the first week of Oil Pulling. Karen believes that Oil Pulling is one of *"God's Miracles."*

Teeth Sensitivity and Cracked Feet Healed
Susan, Australia
After only a few weeks of Oil Pulling, Susan confirms her chronic sensitive teeth condition is now gone and her teeth have become whiter. She also advised the underside of her toes which previously had cracked, dry skin were healed within 2 days of Oil Pulling.

Hemorrhoids and Bad Breath Cleared Up
Lawrence, Texas
Lawrence confirms that his 2 years of chronic bad breath cleared up after only 3 days of Oil Pulling. Also, after only 4 days, his chronic case of hemorrhoids began shrinking with the itching and discharge being almost gone. Lastly, Lawrence asserts his sinuses have cleared, and he now has a decreased desire for cigarettes.

Dental Surgery Averted
Kathie, Oregon
Kathie suffered from multiple pockets and gaps between her teeth and her gums.

Her gums had been inflamed and bleeding for a long time. Her Dentist suggested surgery to remove the loose teeth. She found out about Oil Pulling and decided to try it.

After a few days, Kathie felt an improvement in her gums. After 3 months, her gums were very much improved and looked healthy. Her loose teeth had tightened up and also her teeth looked whiter. The cracked skin on the heels of her feet were almost healed along with having a reduction in her overall aches and pains. Prior to Oil Pulling, Kathie had difficulty climbing the stairs without pain, but she now affirms that pain also is gone.

Kathie loves that Oil Pulling is very inexpensive and simple to do. She declares, *"although it may seem like an odd thing to do, it's fantastic!"*

NEXT ACTION:
 "Follow the Recipe,"
   ...1,2,3...

1. Buy Yourself a Good Quality Oil...
Since you are in fact going to be spitting it down the drain, I suggest getting Kirkland brand Unrefined Coconut Oil from Cosco because it is good tasting and costs only $14 for 84 ounces. You can buy it in-store or online at Cosco.com.
Reminder from Chapter 1:
Since you should also be eating Coconut Oil every day...
You can certainly use the *Kirkland brand Unrefined Coconut Oil* for eating and cooking as well as for Oil Pulling. I also highly recommend *Tropical Traditions Gold Label Virgin Coconut Oil* for eating found at Healthytraditions.com. Although it is more expensive, I find it has a more buttery taste and also has the highest ORAC* rating of all the

Coconut Oils I have researched. *(*ORAC=Oxygen Radical Absorption Capacity, i.e., Antioxidant Capacity)*

2. Oil Pull for 20 Minutes Every Day / How to…

I suggest you keep a small container of Coconut Oil in your bedroom, so that first thing in the morning when you awake, before you do ANYTHING…

- Put 1 or 2 teaspoons of Oil in your mouth & <u>note what time it is.</u>
- Swish the oil around in your mouth, back and forth through the teeth, as you do with mouthwash.
- After 20 minutes, spit it out into the toilet, sink or into the trash can.
- Brush your teeth or rinse your mouth afterwards.
- Give yourself a hand!

3. Practice Oil Pulling 20 minutes every day to achieve and maintain optimal results.

Important:

Once you put the Oil into your mouth, don't just sit there staring at the clock
…Start your day!
By the time you make the bed, get dressed, comb your hair and check your email, that 20 minutes will have passed very quickly.

- It was proven that Oil Pulling for LESS than 20 minutes does NOT work. So, no cheating on the timing! (…I'm watching you…)

Fine Points…

- *Try putting a small amount of Oil (1-2 teaspoons) into your mouth at first, to learn what amount is comfortable for you. <u>Remember that the amount of oil is NOT supposed to fill your mouth</u>, because you will be making saliva during this process which will be adding volume.*

- *Until you get used to Oil Pulling, I would keep a small cup nearby in case you have to cough or sneeze during the process; you can spit the oil into the cup if needed. If this occurs, then simply add oil again to your mouth and "resume" the timing to the full 20 minutes. You do NOT have to start the timing all over again.*

- *In the beginning, you may feel some mucus form at the back of your throat and you feel like coughing. Then just spit oil into a cup. Clear your throat and put that oil or new oil (doesn't matter) back into your mouth and resume timing.*

- *The Oil will be clear when it goes into your mouth but should be milky white when it comes out as it will be filled with a multitude of microbes that have been vacuumed out of your mouth.*

Now guess what…?

You have just mastered one of the oldest, easiest, most potent Holistic Healing and Detox practices on the planet…!

…Yay for you!

Chapter Five

Hydrogen Peroxide
Nature's Unsung Hero

The Goal of this chapter is to reveal to you that *Food Grade Hydrogen Peroxide (H2O2)* is a powerful way to raise the Oxygen level of your body so that microbes cannot take root and breed inside you. Pretty simple. The most important takeaway from this chapter is as follows:

- *Disease and infections thrive in a Low Oxygen body.*

- *Hydrogen Peroxide is an Oxygen Therapy which immediately raises the oxygen level of the body, making it an adverse environment for the breeding of disease-causing microbes.*

- *Properly diluted Food Grade Hydrogen Peroxide is safe to ingest.*

- *It has the Generally Regarded as Safe "GRAS" approval of FDA.*

Cavanaugh, (2008).*The One Minute Cure*;
Dr. Edward C. Rosenow, Mayo Clinic;
William Campbell Douglas, (1990). *Hydrogen Peroxide Medical Miracle*.

Oxygen: Our Life Force...

As everyone knows, we can survive weeks without food, days without water but only minutes without oxygen. It is the most essential and abundant element in our body, required for all vital functions. Our body is composed of approximately 65% oxygen. Most of that is in the form of water, H2O. From the air that we breathe, only 15% oxygen is absorbed into the blood. So, the question is, *how can we safely raise and maintain our oxygen levels?*

Although Essential Oils do raise your oxygen level (*Chapter 2*), properly diluted Food Grade Hydrogen Peroxide brings a more immediate infusion and a higher level of Oxygenation to the entire body.

- *Hydrogen Peroxide is simply 2 parts Hydrogen + 2 parts Oxygen = H2O2.*

- *Inside the body, Hydrogen Peroxide breaks down into simple oxygen and water.*

Is Hydrogen Peroxide Therapy Safe ...?

Approximately 10 Million people have been successfully treated with Hydrogen Peroxide therapy by over 10,000 European Doctors and Naturopaths for over 80 years.

So right about now you are thinking, *"Isn't Hydrogen Peroxide that stuff my mom puts in her hair dye to color her hair?"* The answer is Yes and No.

- *Basically, there are 2 categories of Hydrogen Peroxide (H2O2):*
Food Grade and Non-Food Grade.

VERY IMPORTANT:

- *ONLY properly diluted Food Grade H2O2 is safe for ingestion*

- *Even Food Grade H2O2 MUST be properly diluted before ingesting.*

- *The Non-Food Grade H2O2 should NEVER be ingested.*

Non-Food Grade H2O2 is mainly the 3% version that is used for cuts and scrapes and is found in drugstores. The 20% Non-Food Grade H2O2 is usually used for mixing with hair dye and can be found in a Beauty Supply store.

Oxygen Therapy:
Long List of Scientific Verification and History of Use...

In 1783, Dr. Caillens, a French Physician recorded the curing of a Tuberculosis Patient by having her inhale Oxygen daily. His success was recorded in the *Gazette de Sante.*

In 1820, Dr. Daniel Hill was a surgeon who promoted the use of Oxygen Therapy. He cited it having been successful in the treatment of epilepsy, hydrocephalus, scrophula (a condition caused by Tuberculosis bacteria) and nervous disorders.

There have been a vast amount of studies done on the healing effects of H2O2 dating back to 1886, when a Dr. Demarquay administered H2O2 to test animals to discover their blood turned a very bright red from this immediate infusion of extra Oxygen.

In 1888, Dr. P.L. Cortelyou reported H2O2 therapy was successful in the treatment of nose and throat diseases.

Specifically, he recorded using a nasal spray of H_2O_2 to cure Diphtheria.

In 1916, Stebbing and Turnicliffe administered H_2O_2 intravenously to humans and discovered it rendered *"therapeutic results."*

During World War I, H_2O_2 was used intravenously to treat pneumonia. In 1920, H_2O_2 was used to combat an epidemic of pneumonia which was killing off soldiers in India. This pneumonia had an 80% mortality rate. Doctors T.H. Oliver and Dr. Cantab recorded that they started treating *only the hopeless cases* with H_2O_2. *To their surprise, it saved 50% of their terminal patients.*

In 1940, Dr. Sing discovered that intravenous H_2O_2 kept test subject dogs alive for 16 minutes...without any air going into their lungs...(read that again.)

Dr. Charles Farr also performed in-depth studies on H_2O_2. After analyzing blood samples both before and after H_2O_2 infusion, he found that even the venous blood sample (taken from the veins) had been successfully infused with extra oxygen. This infusion of oxygen profoundly turned even the venous blood so vividly red that the lab technicians insisted the received sample must have come from an artery.

In London, the Middlesex Hospital Medical School Found that H_2O_2 therapy was also effective in the treatment of Malaria.

The success of Oxygen Therapy had become so well known that in the1940s, Father Richard Willhelm created the "Educational Council for Hydrogen Peroxide" (ECHO). His intention was to educate people on the effectiveness of H_2O_2 therapy which included his own records of successful treatments on skin diseases, polio, bacterial infections and mental illness. He established a non-profit organization as a teaching tool for proper dosages and usage of H2O2. Unfortunately, he was swamped by the birth of the prescription drug era, where all focus was then diverted.

In the 1950s, Dr. Reginald Holman performed an experiment where he added 45% H2O2 to the drinking water of laboratory rats who had cancerous tumors. He recorded that within 60 days, those cancerous tumors disappeared.

At the University of North Carolina, Dr. Paul Cummings taught Dental surgery. Subsequently, he learned about H2O2 therapy and used it to treat gum disease with amazing success. *Applying H2O2 therapy, he asserts he achieved a 98% success rate on the treatment of 1,000 patients with gum disease.*

Even Dr. Edward C. Rosenow of the world famous Mayo Clinic had published 450 papers on the use of H2O2 as a successful treatment for a plethora of diseases and disorders. Sadly, his extensive research seemed to have followed the path of many newly discovered natural cures, which is to say, his findings were generally swept under the rug of traditional medicine.

- *The purpose of this chapter is NOT to advise you to run down and get an IV of H2O2. We will be discussing several applications of H2O2 that are quite simple and far less invasive.*

The point of this long litany of evidentiary results is to simply alert you to the fact that, even in dire circumstances, the profound healing effect of H2O2 on the body has been well documented for about 230 years.

Surprise #1: Your Body MAKES H2O2...

As you probably already know, your immune system sends out *killer soldiers* to attack the many microbes that invade our body. These biological troops are called *Leukocytes* otherwise known as white blood cells. By making a mixture of oxygen and hydrogen, a type of white blood cell called a *granulocyte produces H2O2 and uses it to simply engulf and exterminate the invading bacteria. (How awesome is our body?)* This action is called a *respiratory burst.* Without the use of our body's *homemade H2O2,* the human race would have succumbed to common illnesses long, long ago.

Simply put, maintaining an optimal level of oxygen in the body is key to prevailing over pathogens, infections and disease. The body also utilizes H2O2 to perform vital functions including the metabolism of proteins, fats, carbohydrates, minerals, vitamins, as well as to empower the body's Immune System and brain function.

Surprise #2: There is H2O2 in Breast Milk...
(Did I not previously mention that God knows what He's doing ...?)

After what you just learned in the above paragraph, you can now guess why *breastfed babies are historically stronger, healthier, more robust and have much less sickness and allergies than babies that are not breastfed. The Colostrum (first milk) is especially high in H2O2*, meeting the crucial needs of a newborn baby having an underdeveloped immune system. It is the H2O2 plus the *Medium Chain Fatty Acids (Good Fat)* in breast milk that *strengthen and build the infant's fragile and underdeveloped immune system,* while also protecting the baby from common infections. *Breast Milk is God's Secret Recipe for Baby Protection. It is the infant's first line of defense against all invading pathogens including viruses, bacteria, parasites and yeast.*

How H2O2 is such a Powerful Healer and Preventative...

- *Inside the body, H2O2 breaks down into simple OXYGEN and WATER.*

- *Most microbes can NOT live or breed in a HIGH OXYGEN environment.* So, increasing the oxygen level in your body is a simple yet profound preventative and healing modality.

Says Who...?

Says Dr. Otto Warburg, *who won the 1931 Nobel Prize in Physiology for proving that all Viruses and most Bacteria are unable to live or breed in a HIGH OXYGEN environment.* He confirmed that raising the body's oxygen level not only exterminates pathogens but also stimulates and strengthens the Thyroid and Immune System.

To put it another way: almost all microbes are anaerobic, including Cancer. This means they *require a LOW OXYGEN or a NO OXYGEN environment to live and breed.* Dr. Warburg's discovery was twofold: Firstly, that Toxins, Bacteria, Viruses, and Pathogens *cannot live in a High Oxygen environment.* Secondly, he proved that *Cancer thrives in Low Oxygen or No Oxygen at the cellular level.* Both of these revelations were life changing discoveries. His

225

findings asserted that *"if a cell is deprived of just 35% of its Oxygen for 48 hours, it may become cancerous, as the main cause of cancer is insufficient Oxygen at the cellular level."*
 (Warburg, 1931)

The19th century "Father of Pathology" Dr Rudolph Virchow confirmed Pathogens seek weakened (low Oxygen) cells where they can multiply, *like mosquitoes seek stagnant water to breed.*

- *Almost 100 years of research results have concluded that almost all Toxins, Viruses, Bacteria and Disease-causing microorganisms are oxidized (killed) by contact with Oxygen and cannot effectively breed in a High Oxygen environment.*

- *Cancer cells die in the presence of oxygen.*

Simple Science Says...
The Baylor University Group performed an incredibly successful study in 1964, which was properly ignored by the medical community. At that time, the traditional way of Oxygenating the body was by way of using a Hyperbaric Chamber. A Hyperbaric Chamber is an enclosed tube or chamber large enough for the patient to lie down inside. By increasing the pressure inside this chamber, Oxygen is forced into the patient's body tissues. This treatment was very expensive and not without risks. Dr. Finney and his colleagues determined that infusing H2O2 directly into the patient's blood vessels would be more immediately effective, safe, and inconsequential in cost.

It was discovered that *once in the bloodstream, H2O2 breaks down into Oxygen in 1/10 of a second*.

It was further proven that the degree of saturation of the blood was much greater than could be achieved with the Hyperbaric Chamber. When delivered directly into the blood vessels, *H2O2 increased the patients' oxygen level 4x more than the Hyperbaric Chamber and was infinitely faster*. The final and most important recorded discovery was that there was *no negative side effect* to the patient.

Dr. Finney's team then performed extensive testing on patients with severe arteriosclerosis. *Half the patients were treated by dripping the H2O2 directly into the clogged arteries*. The other half of the group were *not treated* with H2O2. Much later, after these test subjects had died, autopsies were performed to learn if there was any difference in the arteries of the two groups. *The results were astonishing. They found that the plaque buildup had been completely dissolved in the arteries of the Patients treated with H2O2.*

To improve breathing for his Patients with Emphysema, Dr. Kurt Donsbach recorded that he instructed them to put 1 oz of 35% *Food Grade H2O2* into a vaporizer near the patient's bed and to run it all night.

Getting to the Heart of the Matter...

The Baylor University Group surged forward with another study in 1962-1966 regarding *cardiac resuscitation with H2O2*. During a heart attack, the heart beats wildly and erratically. Because of this sudden state of Hypoxia (lack of Oxygen), most heart attack victims die within hours of the infarction (obstructed blood supply to the heart). It was *discovered that H2O2 had a revitalizing effect on the heart, causing it to beat with regularity and vigor.* This study confirmed that H2O2 slowed down erratic heartbeat and substantially lowered high blood pressure.

The Baylor Group also performed an extensive experiment with lab animals by obstructing their ability to breathe. Without treatment these test animals would develop cardiac arrest and die in about 5-10 minutes. *But when H2O2 was injected into their arteries, the test animals lived for 2 hours...without breathing.*

(I'm not happy either about how they did animal testing all those years ago, but let's try to focus on the results.)

Next the coronary arteries of test animals were clamped off, stopping the blood supply to their heart. Normally this would cause death by cardiac arrest within 5-10 minutes. But when *H2O2 was injected into the peripheral blood vessels, the animals' heartbeat and blood pressure returned to normal. Finally, it was discovered that even the simple action of just dripping the H2O2 onto the heart muscle saved the animals from cardiac arrest and death.*

Finney, et al. (1967). *Ann. NY Academy of Science.*

In Scientific terms it has been documented: *"Myocardial asemia (lack of Oxygen to the heart) is often dramatically reduced by H2O2, while ventricular fibrillation (chaotic heartbeat) has been found to be completely relieved by the emergency use of H2O2."* (Urshel,1965)

"Gimme the Short Version..."
How did H2O2 prevent Cardiac Arrest from lack of Oxygen...?

228

- *Inside the body, H2O2 breaks down into OXYGEN and WATER in 1/10 of a second, providing what the heart needs to resume normal function.*

How does H2O2 help Heal or Prevent Infection and Disease...?

- *Food Grade H2O2 immediately infuses oxygen into the body. Most pathogens cannot live or breed in a High Oxygen Environment.*

Do I Need to Run Out and Get an I.V....?
Big NO.

- **You do NOT need an intravenous injection to benefit from H2O2. This method is only done in hospitals under dire circumstances and for dire health conditions**.

How do I Safely Use H2O2...?

Because Food Grade H2O2 is so compatible with our blood, it can be absorbed by our body in 3 very simple ways:

1. *Put 5 drops of 12% Food Grade H2O2 into a 10-16 oz of bottled or filtered water to drink.*

2. *Dilute 12% Food Grade H2O2 down to a 3% solution and put it into a clean empty nasal spray bottle. To make a 3% solution, use a 4:1 ratio of water to 12% H2O2.*

3. *Pour 1/2 cup of 12% Food Grade H2O2 into a warm bath and soak for at least 20 minutes.*

Who Says You Can Safely Ingest Food Grade H2O2...?

Dr. Edward C. Rosenow, a renowned Scientist from the world-famous Mayo Clinic, is reputed to be the first to suggest ingesting Food Grade H2O2 orally. He published 450 papers on H2O2 therapy.

In his book *The One-Minute Cure*, Madison Cavanaugh advises a detailed and proven healing regimen of ingesting H2O2 in filtered water.

Dr. William Campbell Douglas also recommends taking 10 drops of 3% Food Grade H2O2 3x a day in his book *Hydrogen Peroxide, Medical Miracle.*

Lastly, *the FDA classifies Food Grade H2O2 as safe to ingest (GRAS) at low dosages.*

- *It MUST be Food Grade H2O2 and it MUST be properly DILUTED.*

Why Do the Pharmaceutical Companies Say No...? Because H2O2 is a naturally occurring substance that can NOT be PATENTED.

The Pharmaceutical industry sells over a Trillion (with a "T") dollars a year worth of antibiotics, heart drugs, blood pressure drugs, you-name-it-we-got-it drugs all day every day. *Prescription drugs are Big Business.* So why in the world would Big Pharma support the use of a natural inexpensive substance that will kill pathogens, clear your arteries and strengthen your heart? They would be shooting themselves in the foot...*(and then writing themselves a prescription for it.)*

The American Medical Association, the FDA, and the Pharmaceutical Companies are united in upholding and protecting their existing protocols. To clarify, we are certainly grateful for the dedicated doctors who are diligently at our hospital bed in time of need. The point being made here is that it's *not their fault that no all-natural preventions or cures are taught to them in Medical School.* As a result of this, *treatments that are unfamiliar to your Doctor will in all likelihood be rejected by your Doctor.*

Dr. Paul Saladino advises he studied for 4 years at College of William and Mary as a Chemistry Major and Pre-Med., plus 2 years at George Washington University, plus 4 years at the University of Arizona, followed by 4 years of practicing as a P.A. in Cardiology and lastly, 4 years at the University of Washington. He is Board Certified in Psychiatry and Functional Medicine.

- *Dr. Saladino confirms that, throughout all his extensive schooling, NONE of these institutions for Medical training required a course in Nutrition; nor did any of them teach how to "find and treat the root cause" of sickness and disease. He affirms he was never trained to treat and rebalance the entire body, i.e., Holistic Healing.*

This alarming realization triggered him to launch his own, well-known crusade to teach *whole body health through nutrition.* Currently, he is continuing his in-depth research on the direct connection between nutrition biochemistry and chronic disease. He is now a Board-Certified Physician Nutrition Specialist.

The above information explains why a conventional physician's orientation is to *treat the symptoms of a disease and not the cause.* As a result, many patients seek Holistic Practitioners who are trained in treating and regaining the health and balance of the entire body.

Death by Prescription Drugs…

- *In cases of long-term use, more prescription drugs usually need to be prescribed to counteract the side effects of the original prescriptions.*

- *In a 2003 Report to Congress, it was revealed that drug interaction and side effects were the THIRD leading cause of death in the U.S. At that time, this was equal to deaths by Cancer*
.

As advised in Chapter 2, my Mother had a very bad case of shingles. The root cause was the Chickenpox Virus. This outbreak occurred each year for 3 years, each time occurring after she received a flu shot. Her Doctor prescribed Vioxx. Why, I don't know. Because the medical industry knows no drugs can kill a virus. I called our Pharmacist who confirmed to my Mother that, in fact, *"no prescription drug can kill a virus."* The Vioxx caused my Mother to have intense joint pain and a distended abdomen; but did nothing to the shingles. *So, why was she given this toxic ineffective drug? Because it was recommended for this purpose by the drug manufacturer. It was a $200 prescription. Understand?*

You will recall from *Chapter 2* that my Mother's Shingles were cured by applying 1 drop each of *Essential Oils of Clove, Lavender, Oregano and Melaleuca,* 3x a day for 6 days. *(Definition of cured = it disappeared and never returned.)*

As advised, a few years later I saw on TV that a Class Action Lawsuit was initiated against the makers of VOIXX because it proved to cause a very *high amount of heart attack*s in its users. It was reputed that this deadly side effect

232

was known by the manufacturer but kept undisclosed to the public. Editor of the *Lancet,* a world famous Medical Journal, assessed that this catastrophe was an *"astonishing failure"* on the part of the drug's manufacturer and a *"lethal weakness" in the FDA.*

(Dr. Richard Horton, *The Lancet*)

H_2O_2 is considered to be a broad spectrum healing modality, meaning it treats a wide range of sickness and disease. Even better news is that *it positively impacts your entire body by delivering an infusion of life-giving, microbe-killing oxygen to every single cell.* No prescription is going to do that.

Modern medicine already uses Oxygen Therapy. When you are admitted to the hospital, you are many times given an oxygen breathing device. For MS and Cancer treatment, popular drugs like Interferon and Verteporfin have had some success in shrinking cancer cells *by using a roundabout way of raising oxygen levels in those cells.* It is well known that oxygen treatment has a powerful healing effect on the body, even in dire conditions. Yet it is highly unlikely that a doctor would advise you to spray a simple 3% solution of Food Grade H_2O_2 in your nostrils to help clear up a sinus infection, or just add 5 drops of 12% Food Grade H_2O_2 to a glass of water and drink it each day *to prevent* most sickness.

- **The point here is NOT to discredit our good medical community for not usually being a source of Holistic Healing, but to awaken your awareness that Natural Healing is simply not their orientation.**

"What Happened with Pop's Feet...?"

Pop was 89 years old and living back East with my Family. When I came out to visit him, I observed his feet were quite frankly unrecognizable as feet. They were a thick-skinned grayish white with dark fungus in his misshapen toenails. They looked like dead, fossilized dinosaur feet that someone dug up from the backyard.

I was only visiting for 2 weeks, so I started an immediate treatment as follows:

I put 1/4 cup of 35% Pure Food Grade H2O2 in a large foot bath basin containing warm water. I had Pop soak his feet in this for an hour each day. Thereafter, I dried his feet and massaged them with raw Coconut Oil mixed with 4 drops each of Eucalyptus and Melaleuca Essential Oils.

Day by day, his feet became pinker and pinker. Within a week, they actually resembled feet again. The toenails did not regain their proper shape but became much clearer. The Podiatrist couldn't believe the difference he saw and asked what we did to revitalize Pop's feet.

Please note that these daily oxygen foot baths also served to *Oxygenate Pop's entire body* as the H2O2 was easily absorbed through his feet and circulated throughout his body. *Big Bonus.*

"Tell Us About the Swimming Pool...!"

Once upon a time, I had a big, beautiful swimming pool in my backyard. It had a waterfall and a jacuzzi and one big problem...*it was just a big toxic bath full of health-diminishing CHLORINE!* Research dictates that repeated absorption of chlorine by the body decreases immune function, thyroid function and interferes with proper hormone function. That being said, *do I want my family to be soaking in it every day?*

234

I did some research on healthier alternatives and discovered that we could *sanitize the pool water and prevent algae by swapping out those toxic Chlorine tablets for*
… oh yes, Hydrogen Peroxide (H2O2).

Our pool had 25,000 gallons of water. My research advised this required *an initial dose* of 6 gallons of pure 35% Food Grade H2O2. Thereafter, I only had to add about 1 gallon of H2O2 per month all summer to keep the water crystal clear and clean. The only other additive I used was 2 oz per month of a Copper algaecide. Copper is a trace mineral which is also beneficial to the body.

Were the results successful…?
Let me tell you, the water was so clean, so soft, so crystal clear…I was in heaven. I realize it may sound a bit crazy to say the water was "soft" but in fact, the water felt like liquid silk. Each time my family went into the pool, we were getting a *Spa Bath of Oxygen.* Once inside the pool, thousands of tiny bubbles covered our skin as *our body naturally and easily absorbed extra oxygen instead of toxic chlorine.*

At that time, I used to swim laps in the pool for exercise. Usually, I couldn't exceed 5 laps before having muscle fatigue. *But the very first day I put the H2O2 into the pool, I was suddenly able to swim 10 laps! I was amazed at how the H2O2 had quickly absorbed into my body, strengthening my muscles with extra Oxygen, enabling me to literally double my laps.*

I never used any other chemical in our pool after that, because I then knew for certain that our bodies were just drinking in the oxygen. The H2O2 was supporting the function of all cells, tissues and organs, making us stronger and healthier each and every time we got into that pool.

235

How To Sanitize Your Pool with H2O2...

You will need to purchase 3 things: 35% Pure Food Grade H2O2, a good Copper Algaecide and H2O2 test strips.

➢ *You will first need to power wash your pool filter to rid it of all gunk and residual debris, chlorine and dirt.*

➢ Next step is to stop adding any Chlorine, Bromine and other toxic chemicals to your pool. Wait a few days for the sun to burn off the residual chlorine. Use your chlorine test strips to learn when the chlorine level has dropped to almost nothing.

➢ Then, your initial dosage should be *approximately 1 gallon of pure 35% Food Grade H2O2 per each 4,300 gallon of pool water.* Also add 2 ounces copper algaecide.

➢ Be sure to use the H2O2 test strips to check H2O2 level each week. The proper level should be between 50-90 ppm. Add more H2O2 accordingly. Expect to be adding an additonal ½ gallon of H2O2 about every 2 weeks. Copper algaecide to be added once a month (read label for proper dosage for your pool size).

My sister has a 12,000 gallon pool to which we *initially added* 3 gallons of 35% Food Grade H2O2 plus 2 oz Copper algaecide. Depending on the temperature and how many people are using the pool, we added about ½ a gallon of 35% Food Grade H2O2 about every 2 weeks, depending on the test strip readings. We also added 2 oz of pure *Copper Algaecide* to her pool once a month. The results were the same as they were for my pool. *Her pool water was soft, clean, crystal clear and just gently bathed us in health-giving oxygen each time we swam.*

When H2O2 level is good, you will be standing in the pool and looking down at your legs to find they are covered in thousands of tiny white bubbles indicating the oxygen is present and active. *It is recommended that you stay in the pool for at least 20 minutes for your body to well absorb that extra oxygen.*

Now you have achieved an all-in-one clean, disinfected pool plus an Oxygen Spa treatment each time you swim. That's a huge Win-Win.

So Say the Experts...

One of the world's most prominent experts on natural healing is Dr. David G. Williams who applauded the many health-giving benefits of H2O2 in a 4,200-word article. Initially, he was quite skeptical. *But after exhaustive research along with many clinical studies he affirmed he is convinced that H2O2 is a "safe and effective therapy that is readily available, inexpensive and, best of all, it works!"*
(Williams, 2003)

The world-famous *Gerson Institute, Advanced Therapy Clinic* is based upon the lifelong research of Dr. Max Gerson. His results of cancer regression were so successful he wrote a book in 1959 called *A Cancer Therapy: Results of 50 Cases.* After his death, his daughter Charlotte Gerson and Dr. Vickers resumed the application of Gerson's unique healing protocol for the regression of Cancer and other historically fatal diseases, achieving the same extraordinary results.

I bring this to your attention to note that the Gerson Institute incorporates several methods of Oxygen Therapy into their healing protocol for advanced diseases. Their

Protocol includes other components including a strict mostly raw diet and supplements as well.

The takeaway here is that the reputation of the Gerson Clinic is beyond reproach. The Gerson Advanced Disease Therapies have a 60 year history of worldwide success, and they use Oxygen Therapy in their protocols.

Last but certainly not least, is Dr. Christian Bernard. Dr. Bernard is a world-famous Heart Surgeon, renowned for performing the first successful heart transplant surgery in 1967. He attests he recommended H2O2 therapy to his patients as a post-surgery protocol to assist in healing and avert infection. Dr. Bernard disclosed that he was ridiculed by the medical community for this protocol, yet he *continued with it successfully. He even used H2O2 therapy on himself to successfully treat his arthritis and other disorders. He affirmed he was amazed at its efficacy.*

Summing Up the Wisdom ...

H2O2 is considered to be a broad-spectrum healing modality, meaning it treats a wide range of sickness and disease. Even better news is that it positively impacts your entire body by delivering an infusion of life-giving, microbe-killing oxygen to every single cell as it eradicates pathogens. No prescription drug can do that.

H2O2 fights against the breeding of pathogens in the body while invigorating each cell with extra oxygen. This includes brain cells. It has been shown to increase mental focus and improve memory while also increasing stamina and muscle performance.

It is no small thing that a world-famous Heart Surgeon with Dr. Christian Bernard's accolades used H2O2 to achieve healing for himself and also to ensure his patients had successful post-op healing.

We remember that in 1931, Dr. Otto Warburg won the Nobel Prize in Physiology for proving that all Viruses and most Bacteria are unable to live or breed in a HIGH OXYGEN environment. He affirmed that raising the Body's Oxygen level not only exterminates pathogens but also stimulates and strengthens the Thyroid and Immune System. He further proved that Cancer breeds in low-oxygen cells.

In total, it is estimated that approximately 6,100 articles have been recorded in scientific publications on the therapeutic success of H2O2 treatment. There are approximately 15,000 Doctors and Naturopaths in Europe who use or have used Oxygen Therapy to treat over 1 million patients. Here in the U.S., we have only an estimated 500 Doctors and Naturopaths who utilize this amazing therapy.

Dr. William Campbell Douglas. (1990). *Hydrogen Peroxide, Medical Miracle.*

Where to Buy Food Grade 12% H2O2...

Be sure the Product is 12% *PURE FOOD GRADE Hydrogen Peroxide.* Amazon is one source for 12% Food Grade H2O2.

- *Product MUST COME with a small Cobalt Blue glass dropper bottle. This is important* as you will transfer the H2O2 from the big bottle into this small one to then measure the proper amount of drops into your water.

Note: the dropper bottle must be GLASS and DARK COLORED to properly store the H2O2, to protect it from light which will degenerate it, making it less effective.

How To Transfer H2O2 from the Big Bottle into the Small Dropper Bottle...

- *Remove the top of the dropper bottle and put the bottle into the sink.*
- *Wear rubber gloves in case it spills onto your hands.*
- *Use a small funnel to carefully pour the H2O2 into the dropper bottle.*
- *If it overflows a bit, we don't care because it's in the sink isn't it?*
- *Replace bottle top and run water over the bottle before picking it up.*
- *I keep mine in the refrigerator although you only need to keep it in a cool place.*

CAUTION:

- **YOU CAN ONLY INGEST PROPERLY DILUTED FOOD GRADE H2O2.**

NEXT ACTION:
"Follow the Recipe"
...1,2,3...

1. To Drink:

Dilute 12% Pure Food Grade H2O2 *by putting 5 drops into 10-16 oz glass of bottled water and drink on an empty stomach, not with meals.*

- *Best take first thing in the morning before breakfast.*
- *It can be taken anytime of the day but not with food.*

240

- *Can be taken before bed.*

2. Nasal Spray Application:
- ***Must Dilute 12% Food Grade H2O2 down to a 3% solution*** *and put it into a clean empty nasal spray bottle. Put a squirt or 2 into each nostril while inhaling.*

- *To make 3% solution, use a 4:1 ratio of bottled water to 12% Food Grade H2O2.*

3. In Bath:
- *Pour ¼ - ½ cup of 12% Food Grade H2O2 into a ½ bathtub of warm water and soak for at least 20 minutes. This will effectively soothe sore muscles and oxygenate the body.*

For Healthy Gums and Whiter Teeth:
Use a 3% solution of Food Grade H2O2 to rinse mouth or gargle with.

- *Can also put 3% Food Grade H2O2 into a small spritzer bottle to spray onto the toothbrush, then brush teeth.*

- *Can spray a 3% Food Grade H2O2 solution directly onto teeth and gums.*

Other Applications:
- *Can put 25 drops of 12% Food Grade H2O2 into a half gallon of filtered or bottled water and drink it throughout the day or week.*

- *To treat chest congestion, lung infections: Can put 4 oz of <u>12% Food Grade</u> H2O2 into a gallon of water in a vaporizer. Place vaporizer near bed and run it all night.*

- *Can spray <u>3%</u> Food Grade H2O2 solution directly onto acne breakout, bruises, scrapes and cuts.*

- <u>*To make 3% solution, use a 4:1 ratio of bottled water to 12% Food Grade H2O2.*</u>

Be aware of Possible Healing Crises...

As with Oil Pulling, some people may experience slight symptoms when beginning their H2O2 therapy, such as runny nose, headache or a slight skin rash.

Remember this is a *healing crisis which clearly indicates that your body is ridding itself of toxins*. This should pass within a week.

IMPORTANT:

- *I do NOT advise in any chapter of this book that you just suddenly stop taking your medication. In all advised instances of healing, the reduction of medication was gradual.*

- *I can NOT promise that the Holistic Practices in this book will eliminate every medication you are currently taking; but historically, these treatments have proven to be highly successful overall in greatly reducing the need for many prescription medications.*

- *I can NOT promise that the methods outlined in this book will heal every ailment you may have or that it will work exactly the same as it has worked for me.*

- *However...firmly based on the 30 years of successful treatments I have witnessed, I can say that it is exponentially more likely that you will live a healthier life if you properly follow some or most of these Holistic Healing practices, as directed.*

You are the Master Builder of your Health.

WHAT YOU HAVE LEARNED SO FAR:
WHAT THREE THINGS CAN KILL A VIRUS...?
By now you have learned there are three things that can safely kill a virus and most other pathogens:
- ➢ *Unrefined Coconut Oil*
- ➢ *Therapeutic Grade Essential Oils*
- ➢ *Food Grade Hydrogen Peroxide*

You have learned that Oil Pulling "attracts and traps" oral microbes so you can simply expel them from your mouth. This greatly relieves your Immune System and empowers the body to "heal itself."

You have learned that replacing ALL processed oils with unrefined Coconut Oil will strongly prevent type 2 diabetes, restore cell health and increase brain function while killing pathogens and fungus in the body.

IF you have also learned that eliminating "Avoid Foods" for your blood type will protect against inflammation, thick blood and autoimmune disorders ...well then,
... you may go to the head of the Class.

At this point in your journey, you are now well informed on all of these Natural, Whole Body Healing Therapies, which are both powerful and extraordinary.

Use these Holistic Healing Bricks to build yourself a Powerhouse of Wellness.

244

Chapter Six

Are Your Teeth Killing You?

What if I told you…
There are probably one or more toxic pumps in your mouth, streaming pathogens into your bloodstream right now?

What if I told you…
Swollen and bleeding gums are like a big sponge, absorbing microbes from your mouth and passing them into your bloodstream all day, every day?

What if I told you…
There is a way to remedy all of this…?

We already learned in Chapter 4 that most diseases begin in the mouth. Now we will dive into how this happens…*and what you can do about it.*

Let's Talk About Your Pearly Whites…
Your teeth are probably one of the most important yet least understood parts of your body. Teeth are a remarkable work of art. The outer surface which covers each tooth, called the *enamel*, is the hardest tissue in our body. The root, which is the portion of the tooth below the gumline, is covered by a

thinner coving called the *cementum*. Then we have the *dentin*, which is found underneath the enamel and cementum. The term *"Dentist"* was derived from the word *Dentin*. Lastly, deep inside the tooth is the *pulp* which houses the nerves and the blood supply that keeps each tooth alive.

Similar to bones, your teeth are *living tissue*. The enamel is continuously *remineralizing* (getting stronger and harder) or *demineralizing* (getting thinner and weaker) depending on the pH of your mouth. For example, if your mouth becomes continuously acidic (having a low pH) then your enamel thins out and weakens. This is exactly what happens when you regularly drink sodas (yes even diet sodas) which make the mouth acidic. Also, the bacteria in your mouth feed on sugar and, in turn, produce even more acid as a by-product. This acidic environment eats away at the enamel of your teeth, slowly but steadily. Now you know why soda is the perfect superfood for cavities.

How Swollen Gums Cause Sickness Throughout the Body ...

Inflammation or swelling of the gums is known as *Gingivitis,* which is the first stage of gum disease. It is estimated that approximately 80% of the population has stage one Gingivitis. Yet the early symptoms of having swollen or bleeding gums are usually ignored.

Chronic Gingivitis progresses to where the inflamed gums recede, pulling away from the teeth. This creates pockets or gaps around the teeth, giving destructive bacteria and acids access to the root of the tooth. Now, bacteria and toxins have a new place to gather and breed as they attack the tooth below the gumline. Inflammation increases and infection develops. This causes the eventual breakdown of bone and connective tissue which hold the tooth in place.

This Phase is called *Pyorrhea* or *Periodontitis*. Without treatment, the Patient will lose one or more teeth. Worst case scenario, he may also suffer jawbone loss from the unattended infection and chronic inflammation.

When I was a little girl, I vividly remember my grandmother needing to have all her teeth removed because she had *Pyorrhea.* My Mother tried to explain to me that even though Grandmom's teeth looked fine, all her teeth needed to be removed because her *gums were so unhealthy.*

We discussed in Chapter 4 that the mouth harbors 600 different kinds of microbes (bacteria, viruses, toxins). There are *10 Billion microbes (germs)* living quietly in your mouth right now. *They are relatively harmless…as long as they remain in your mouth.*

We learned that any break in the gums or having the *condition of swollen or bleeding gums allow this multitude of microbes to pass through the gums and easily enter the bloodstream.* Once in the bloodstream, these microbes target other areas of the body causing infection and disease. Please note that these disease-causing pathogens a*re passing through your gums even from Stage 1 of gum disease.* Left unchecked, it simply worsens from there, eventually developing into tooth and gum infections and death of the tooth.

- **All Stages of Gum Disease allow pathogens to pass through the gums into the bloodstream, slowly infecting other areas of the body**.

- **The Center for Disease Control and Prevention affirms that 90% of the population has tooth decay and ⅓ of all adults over the age of 65 have lost all their teeth.**

247

How Infected Teeth Cause Sickness Throughout the Body...

Dr. Bruce Fife refers to our mouth as harboring a "microbial soup" of bacteria, viruses, fungi and parasites. Since our gums are so dense with capillaries, any break in the gum including ulcers will open the access door for these microbes to spread into the bloodstream. Please note *that swollen and bleeding gums have already opened that door...and are holding it open.*

Initially, the bacteria and acids in your mouth eat their way through the *enamel* of the tooth causing what we call a *cavity.* This is Phase 1. Next, the cavity will bore its way into the *dentum*, causing the symptom of tooth sensitivity, receding gums and gaps between teeth and the gums. That is Phase 2. If left unattended, the cavity continues to eat its way into the heart of the tooth, the *pulp*, which is when all the real problems begin. Once the infection invades the pulp of the tooth, it then easily expands into the root. An acute infection or abscess develops. This is Phase 3. By Phase 3, the gums have receded, and you now have a *Toxic Pump* in the root of your tooth. Due to lack of effective treatment, the problem has multiplied. The Patient now has an abscessed tooth, one or more loose teeth and severely infected gums. Without proper treatment the tooth will die, and very often, the surrounding teeth will die also. But that's not the real threat here.

The biggest problem is the one you don't even see:

- **Now that the pulp of the tooth is infected, that tooth has become a "Toxic Pump" flowing a steady stream of bacteria and infection into your bloodstream.**

248

- *Decades of research confirms that oral bacteria travels through the bloodstream from the mouth and attacks various parts and organs of the body.*

- *Most oral microbes are harmless as long as they remain in the mouth; but they wreak havoc on our health once they enter the bloodstream. There they can cause a host of systemic or local infections, inflammation and a myriad of disorders from arthritis to heart disease.*

This centuries-old realization became known as the *"Focal Infection Theory of Disease."* We have learned how for hundreds of years Farmers habitually checked an animal's mouth before buying it, because an *unhealthy mouth indicates current or impending sickness. Centuries ago, it was generally known that an unhealthy mouth eventually turns into a very unhealthy body, for man or beast.*

What Say the Experts…?

Dr Weston A. Price is viewed as the world's leading expert on the profound effects of Oral Health on the body. In 1923, the results of his exhaustive 25-year study was recorded in a 2 volume text called Dental Infections, Oral and Systemic Volume I and Dental Infections and Degenerative Disease Volume II. Within the 1,174 pages of this publication <u>*Dr. Price documented in great detail his proof that almost all diseases begin in the mouth and that disease is primarily the result of Oral Bacteria which has traveled throughout the body*</u>*. Mouth bacteria in other parts of the body have been proven to cause a wide range of diseases including arthritis, endocarditis (heart disease), arteriosclerosis, liver disorders and diabetes.*

Dr. Price worked with a stellar team of 60 scientists including Dr. Charles H. Mayo, President of the Clinical Congress of Surgeons of North America and who also established the famous Mayo Clinic; Dr. Frank Billings, Head of Department of Medicine at University of Chicago; Dr. Victor C. Vaughan, Dean of the Medical Department at University of Michigan and President of the American Medical Association; and Dr. Milton J. Rosenau, Professor of Preventive Medicine and Hygiene at Harvard Medical School. *Let us pause here to realize that after 25 years of research plus reconfirmation by the above All-Star Team of experts, Dr. Price's discovery that disease begins as a result of mouth bacteria has been long accepted as an indisputable medical fact.*

Now, let's use this revelation to our ultimate advantage.

As we learned, Hippocrates the Greek Physician and acclaimed *"Father of Modern Medicine"* preached 2,700 years ago that he could *cure patients of arthritis by simply pulling out their infected teeth*. This discovery is documented in ancient Assyrian and Greek medical Texts. All the way up to the 1900s, it was a widely accepted protocol to pull infected teeth to resolve a plethora of patient disorders. However, when the antibiotics tsunami hit the medical arena, the revised go-to Dental Protocol became: *Leave the infected tooth; and just write a prescription*. Some antibiotics can hold an abscess at bay. But more often than not, once the prescription is finished, the infection flares back up because it is in the pulp of the tooth which cannot be successfully treated with antibiotics.

Root Canal, the Royal Toxic Pump...

By the early 1900s, Dentistry embraced a very popular (and expensive) practice for dealing with severely infected teeth: *Leave the infected tooth in place & just perform a Root Canal.* For those of you that haven't had the pleasure, a root canal is the procedure whereby the infected pulp of the tooth is drilled out, allegedly disinfected and then filled with a rubber-like substance before capping the tooth off.

Dr. Weston Price was the first to discover *that* **_every root canal tooth is still infected_**. *By capping the infected tooth, the toxins are simply directed downward into the jaw and into the bloodstream* **_creating a Toxic Pump_**.

One of his patients had severe arthritis to the point of having deformed joints. Unable to walk, this patient was in a wheelchair for 6 years. Despite the fact that no x-ray showed any sign of infection, Dr. Price insisted that the root canal tooth be pulled. The tooth was commercially disinfected then implanted under the skin of a rabbit. After 2 days, the rabbit developed the same crippling arthritis as the patient. In 10 days, that rabbit died from the root canal tooth which was "assumed disinfected" but was, in actuality, was festering all those years in the patient's mouth. What happened to the patient? According to Dr. Price's records, "the Patient had a miraculous recovery" after the root canal tooth was removed. (Price, 1923)

Key Points:
- *No sign of tooth infection showed on the Patient's X-ray. Yet after extraction, _the root canal tooth was so septic_ that in just 2 days it infected the test animal with*

the same disease and same severe symptoms as the Patient.

- *Before being implanted into the rabbit, the extracted root canal tooth was soaked in very strong commercial disinfectants. How did that work out for the rabbit...?*

- *If soaking the extracted tooth in strong commercial disinfectants can NOT rid the tooth of infection, then we know that nothing a Dentist uses in your mouth can "disinfect" that toxic tooth, correct?*

- *Science has confirmed:*
  A root canal tooth is still infected and acts as a Toxic Pump in your mouth.

Dr. Price went on to do hundreds more tests and experiments which reconfirmed that root canal teeth were still extremely infected with disease-causing bacteria. Even after extraction and attempts at commercial-grade disinfection, these teeth caused the *exact same disease in test animals as they did in the patient.* If the patient had ovarian disease, the test rabbit got ovarian disease; if the patient had heart disease, the test rabbit got heart disease; if the Patient had rheumatism, the test rabbit got rheumatism. The same thing happened with phlebitis and even stomach ulcers. Lastly, he recorded *that all previously healthy test animals died within 2 weeks of having a root canal tooth implanted under their skin. The results were both shocking and indisputable:*

- *All root canal teeth are all still infected.*

- *The root canal procedure only serves to turn that tooth into a septic fountain of bacteria and toxins.*

Dr. Edward C. Rosenow led a team of researchers at the world-famous Mayo Clinic performing extensive studies on this oral causation of disease known as *Focal Infection*. His results confirmed those of Dr. Price. This Mayo Clinic study lasted over 20 years and is documented by over 200 scientific reports. It was further discovered that infected root canal teeth also negatively affected blood chemistry, directly impacting migraines, osteoporosis and hormonal imbalance.

"Death and Dentistry"...
Martin H. Fischer, M.D., was a Professor of Physiology at the University of Cincinnati. In 1940, Dr. Fischer wrote the Book *Death and Dentistry,* which compiled *his 40 years of exhaustive research on the oral causation of disease,* including Multiple Sclerosis, asthma, senility, colitis, dermatitis and hypertension, to name a few. Sadly, his revelations and documentation of oral health's impact on the body was quickly drowned by the use of antibiotics flooding most medical protocols around that time.

Finally, in 2000, the U.S. Department of Health and Human Services presented an in-depth report to the Surgeon General which *clearly documented the direct connection between oral health and systemic disease.*

U.S. Dept. of Health and Human Services. (2000). *Oral Health in America: A Report of the Surgeon General.* Rockville, MD.

Nat'l Inst. of Health. (2000). *Dental and Craniofacial Research.*

Hardening of the Arteries from Oral Bacteria...

Streptococcus Sanguis (S. sanguis) is in everyone's mouth and is the main bacteria in dental plaque. *It has been shown that this bacteria is also a major cause of arterial plaque and blood clots. This is because it carries a platelet aggregation protein which has the ability to basically glue blood cells together.* Over the years, more and more blood cells become glued together and the blood thickens. Thick blood becomes sticky and tends to form blood clots. It is these blood clots blocking the arteries to the heart and brain that are the number one cause of heart attack and stroke. This is one reason why almost all elderly patients are on "blood thinners."

- *Research has discovered live oral bacteria in arterial plaque.*
- *It has been shown that the more oral plaque and gum disease you have, the greater the likelihood of you developing arterial plaque.*

When plaque builds up in the arteries, the artery becomes narrower forcing the blood through at higher pressure. This pressure causes tiny tears in the arteries. These tears are efficiently "patched up" by our immune system which creates a biological band-aid made of cholesterol, blood platelets, proteins and calcium. It is the calcium that makes these patches "hard," hence the term, hardening of the arteries.

Oral Health and Heart Disease...

There is a multitude of research evidence on the direct connection between oral bacteria and heart disease. In 1965, it was reported in the *Journal of Periodontal Research* that

254

patients who had existing heart issues were at substantial risk for developing Bacterial Endocarditis a few weeks after having a dental procedure. As advised, this is the main reason Dentists administer an antibiotic to patients with a heart condition before performing a dental procedure.

Does Anyone Here Have a Dog...?

We dog owners are well aware that if our dog's gums and teeth fall into poor health or infection, what does our Vet tell us? He warns us that *poor oral health in our beloved pet can directly and adversely affect their heart health.*

Oral Health and Bone Loss...

Periodontal disease has also been linked to bone loss, specifically the jawbone. However, when oral bacteria travel through the bloodstream to other parts of the body such as hips or joints, it causes localized inflammation. *Localized chronic inflammation degenerates the bone in that area.*

Oral Health and Neurological Disease...

Disturbingly, clinical studies have confirmed that many oral pathogens travel easily along nerve cells. This led to the connection between poor oral health and neurological disorders such as Alzheimer's, Parkinson's Disease and Multiple Sclerosis. A study was performed on 144 patients between the ages of 75 and 98. Results showed that the *greater the amount of tooth decay and gum disease, the higher was the incidence of neurological disease.*

Nakayama, Y., et al. (2004). *Oral Health Conditions in Patients with Parkinson's Disease. J. Epidemial.* McGrother, C.W., et al. (1999). *Multiple Sclerosis, Dental Caries and Fillings. Br Dent J.*, Stein, P.S., et al. (2007).

Tooth Loss, Dementia and Neuropathology Nun Study.
J Am Dent Assoc.

In one of my Wellness classes, I had a student named Patty who had been a Dental Surgical Nurse for 25 years. I was thrilled. I asked her in front of the class to please interject if she hears anything I am teaching that is not accurate as compared to her medical training and 25 years' experience. I asked her to confirm to the class whether or not in fact all root canal teeth are still infected even after the root canal was done. *She unhesitatingly agreed this was true. She further confirmed that root canal teeth are still infected even after the patient has finished their antibiotics and remain infected for the life of the patient. Patty agreed with the experts who attest that the only way to stop the toxic pump is to have the tooth pulled.* You may choose to have an artificial tooth implanted in its place, but either way, you will have stopped the toxins and bacteria from steadily seeping into your body, stealthily wreaking havoc wherever they go.

Many times, disorders and illnesses develop in various parts of the body, and no one knows why. *No one ever suspects it could be coming from their still-infected root canal teeth, which have been flowing toxins into the patient's bloodstream for years.*

- *Oral bacteria can negatively affect your heart, arteries, blood, brain, bones and all other organs and functions of the body.*
- *Every Root Canaled tooth is a septic pump.*

Says Who...?
The Founder of the American Association of Root Canal Specialists (Endodontists), Dr. George E. Meinig,

attests that infected teeth carry their infection deep inside the tiny, microscopic holes in the tooth called tubules. Once the infection has penetrated the tubules, they live there permanently and become impervious to antibiotics and disinfectants. That tooth then becomes a fountain of toxins that travels throughout the body.

George E. Meinig D.D.S. wrote an expose called *The Root Canal Cover-Up.* In his Book, he plainly asserts, "*The underlying problem still exists, <u>there is still live bacteria inside all root canalled teeth</u>. Antibiotics and disinfectants do not get rid of them. No root canal tooth is free from potentially harmful bacteria. It is safer to pull a severely diseased tooth rather than plug it and cap it, forming a breeding ground of decay, sealing in poisons and bacteria that will leak into your bloodstream for the rest of your life.*" (Meinig, 1994)

So says *the Founder and Head of the American Association of Root Canal Specialists*

…that pretty much nailed it for me.

Toxic Lollipops / Silver (Amalgam) Fillings…

According to the FDA, 50% of all silver (amalgam) fillings are made of liquid elementary mercury. With a statement of fact like this from the FDA, I shouldn't have to go any further.

…oh but you know that I will.

In 2021, the FDA posted that all Amalgam (silver) fillings are composed of *50% liquid mercury* with the remaining 50% being a mixture of silver, tin and copper. The mercury is used to bind the other metals together making a putty commonly known as the "filling" for a cavity. The FDA asserts that these amalgam fillings *slowly release low levels of mercury vapor into the mouth and this is also inhaled into the lungs.* Medical history records mercury as having a substantial negative impact on the health of the brain and kidneys. Specifically, the developing brains of young children are more affected by the mercury vapor from amalgam fillings. It has also been proven that mercury from dental fillings is *bioaccumulative*, meaning *it slowly builds up in the tissues and organs of our body, over time.*

"Mad as a Hatter"...

The poisonous effect that mercury has on the human body has been known for hundreds of years. If you ever read *Alice in Wonderland*, you are familiar with the term *"He is mad as a Hatter."* This colloquialism spawned from 18th century Hat Makers who used *mercury paste* to make their hats. By way of inhalation and absorption through their fingers, the toxic mercury passed into the Hat Makers' bodies, accumulating in their brain and causing many of them to have neurological disorders, i.e., they went mad. *"Mad as a Hatter."*

Acknowledging that mercury was a poisonous substance, the American Society of Dental Surgeons *banned the use of mercury* fillings in the early 1800s, calling it *"Unethical."* At that time, gold foil was the mode of choice for tooth repair. However, gold was expensive and challenging to melt. Mercury is liquid. It was discovered that when mixed with the other metals, it made a soft, moldable putty, ideal for plugging holes in the tooth. Since mercury was much cheaper and easier to work with, most Dentists continued to use it. By 1856, the American Society of Dental Surgeons was nullified.

In 1859, the National Dental Association was formed, later called the American Dental Association (ADA). They promoted the use of amalgam fillings, alleging it was safe.

In the 1920s, a Scientist named Alfred Stock, Ph.D. resurrected the alarming impact amalgam fillings have on overall health. He himself had developed a neurological disorder and suspected it was his amalgam fillings that were the cause. *After having all his amalgam fillings removed, he recorded that he had an almost immediate recovery.* He went on to further demonstrate that mercury gas in fact *continually emanates from amalgam fillings*. He authored many scientific publications on this discovery. However, his work was generally shunned by the Dental community.

- **Once his silver fillings were removed, Scientist Alfred Stock attests that he immediately recovered from his neurological disorder.**

Alfred Stock, Ph.D. (1926). *Dangerousness of Mercury Vapor*

In the 1960s, multiple Researchers reconfirmed that toxic mercury vapor is continuously released from an amalgam filling. Confronted with overwhelming evidence of this, the ADA admitted this was true but alleged that it only happens for a short time after filling is placed. This was disproved by studies which confirmed *that the longer an amalgam filling is in the mouth, the LESS mercury it contains, as it continuously leaks out of the tooth and into the mouth.*

It was discovered that older fillings have *only 10-20% remaining* of their original mercury content. Now we clearly know where the other 80-90% went. Repeated experiments showed conclusively that the mercury in fillings leaks into the body until there is almost no more mercury left in that filling.

- *When analyzed using gas chromatography, it was discovered that amalgam filled teeth from a 10-year-old cadaver still emitted Mercury vapor.*

Berlin, M.H., et al. (1969). Mechanism of Mercury Resorption in the Lung.
Archives of Environmental Health.
Kudak, F.N. (1965). Absorption of Mercury from the Respiratory Tract in Man.
Acta Pharmacology Toxicology,
Svare, C.W., et al. (1981). The Effects of Dental Amalgams on Mercury Levels.
Journal of Dental Research.

Autoimmune Disease
When the Body Attacks Itself...

Our bodies have an amazingly diligent Immune System. Continuously, it sends out white blood cells, like soldiers whose sole mission is to search out and attack any intruders in the body. These soldiers tirelessly seek to confirm that every cell they assess has the *unique Cell Code which is specific to each one of us.* This *Cell Code* identifies as *"Self"* and therefore *"Safe."* When mercury enters the body, it attaches to our cell membranes and thereby *alters the Cell Code* from *"Self"* to *"Non-Self."* *This result causes the Immune System Soldiers to attack it.*

In effect, mercury triggers our Immune System to attack what it perceives as a foreign invader, unaware that our own healthy cell lies beneath.

The Short Version:
- *Heinz et al. attests that the saliva in our mouth reacts with the Mercury vapor to form methylmercury. Research results prove that this*

highly toxic form of Mercury contributes to many neurological and autoimmune disorders, including Multiple Sclerosis.

- *Mercury can alter our cell code to appear as a "foreign cell." This triggers our Immune System to unknowingly attack our own cells, causing Autoimmune disorders.*

"Solving the MS Mystery"...

Hal Huggins, D.D.S. solidified the concrete connection between Multiple Sclerosis and amalgam fillings. He declared he would write a book only after he has studied 1,000 cases of MS, as related to patients with amalgam fillings. True to his word, Dr. Huggins thereafter authored the Book, Solving the MS Mystery. **Dr. Huggins' research confirmed that mercury poisoning promotes a plethora of neurological and autoimmune disorders** *such as Grave's Disease, MS, Lupus, Rheumatoid Arthritis, Addison's Disease and ALS.*

Huggins, H. (1993). *It's All in Your Head: The Link Between Mercury Amalgams and Illness.* Avery Publishing.

Heinz V., et al. (1983). Methylation of Mercury from Dental Amalgam.

Scandinavian Journal of Dental Research.

The Gerson Institute for Healing:

The world-famous Gerson Institute has a long and stellar history of successfully healing dire cases of disease for over 60 years. *The Gerson Institute advises it will not even begin its healing protocols until the patient has ALL ROOT CANAL TEETH REMOVED FIRST. This bold requirement asserts quite clearly that the only way to achieve*

261

optimal healing of the entire body is to first remove the Toxic Pumps from your mouth. How well they know that there is little point in trying to heal the patient if *septic teeth* are still in place, pumping toxins continually into their body. That patient would be swimming upstream in the river of healing.

Is It Safe to Have Nickel in my Mouth…?
That would be a No.

Nickel is often used along with porcelain in dental appliances such as crowns and bridgework. Those which are called "Chrome Crowns" are actually composed of stainless steel and *nickel.* Although not as bad as mercury, nickel is also a heavy metal which is toxic to the body. Nickel appliances can be replaced with those made with gold and porcelain instead.

To give you a reference point of metal toxicity, please note the following 2018 "*maximum contaminant limist*" set by the Environmental Protection Agency (EPA) for our drinking water:

- *Max limit for cyanide in drinking water is 0.2 ppm (parts per million)*

- *Max limit for nickel in drinking water is only 0.1 ppm (parts per million)* <u>*The EPA judges nickel to have twice the toxicity of Cyanide*</u>*, that is, it takes only half the amount of nickel to be considered toxic.*

- *But the winner is… mercury.*
  Alarmingly more toxic than cyanide, the maximum contaminant limit for mercury in drinking water is set at a mere 2 parts per BILLION (yes that's with a "B").

The FDA considers anything over this minute amount to be toxic to the human body.

The World Health Organization (WHO) declares that mercury, specifically methylmercury emitted by amalgam fillings, is most toxic. It negatively affects the immune system, genetic and enzyme system, interferes with brain and nervous system functions, impairs taste and sight, hinders the neurological development of children, including behavior and speech development.

By now you should be asking yourself,
"Should I continue to allow mercury fillings
to reside in my mouth?"

Testimonials...
Fife, B. (2008). *Oil Pulling Therapy.*

Migraines healed...
Dr. Bruce Fife affirms in his Book that many Patients have had an almost immediate recovery from chronic diseases and disorders by simply having the *root cause* (pardon the pun) removed from their mouth. His own wife had suffered with severe chronic migraines for years. There was no relief for her in any medications. But when she had all her amalgam (silver) fillings removed, *her headaches vanished almost immediately and had not returned for 10 years,* up to the writing of his book.

Jaw Rot...

Alice was only 30 years old when she had her root canal done. Although she complained for years to multiple Dentists that the tooth still hurt, her complaints were ignored. At the age of 55, Alice finally found a Dentist who agreed with her insistence that her root canal tooth be pulled. When it was finally pulled, she attests that "*a river of pus ran down her chin.*" The tooth next to the extracted one died and later, another tooth. She had to have several teeth extracted from the same area of the mouth. Finally, it was discovered that the infection from her root canal tooth had spread into her jawbone. *This went unobserved for decades.* As a result, Alice now suffers from severe jawbone deterioration. *All this developed from the infection of her original root canal tooth, which had remained invisibly infected for 25 years.*

Multiple Ailments Cured...

A 61-year-old Patient named Frank had endured chronic headaches, ear infections, joint pain, severe eczema, stomach ulcers, irregular heartbeat and tremors in his right arms. Frank was a sick pup. In his mouth was found 6 amalgam filled teeth and 2 bridges containing nickel. *His savvy Dentist suggested removing the amalgam filling and also replacing the nickel bridge with one made from gold and porcelain.*

Patient felt increasingly better day by day. After only a few short weeks, all his previous symptoms had dramatically decreased. After a few months, Frank reported that all his symptoms had vanished, even the severe Eczema.

Neurological Disorder Vanished...

In the 1920s, a Scientist named Alfred Stock, PhD. was researching the profound negative impact that amalgam fillings have one's overall health. He himself had developed a neurological disorder and suspected it was his amalgam fillings that were the cause. *After having all his amalgam fillings removed, he recorded that he had an almost immediate recovery. (Stock, 1926)*

Crippling Arthritis Healed…

Dr. Weston A. Price affirms that one of his patients had severe arthritis to the point of having deformed joints. Unable to walk, this patient was in a wheelchair for 6 years. Despite the fact that *no x-ray showed any sign of infection,* Dr. Price insisted that the root canal tooth be pulled. According to Dr. Price's records, *"the Patient had a miraculous recovery" after the root canal tooth was removed. This proved that the Patient's severe arthritis was the result of her infected root canal tooth which had been festering in her mouth and flowing toxins into her body, for years.*

What Can I Do To Maximize My Oral Health…?

Let's begin with a short recap of how to avert dental disaster in the first place.

Practicing *Oil Pulling* (*Chapter 4*) for 20 minutes every day is a very simple but powerful method of lowering the *toxic load* of pathogens in your mouth, day by day. We have already seen many *Oil Pulling* testimonials regarding the healing of swollen gums, and loose teeth and how it is effective at reversing stage one Gingivitis. *However, neither this practice nor any other method of healing can completely overcome a toxic pump in your mouth.*

Remember our Motto…?
To achieve optimal health you must first:

265

- **"Plug the Holes in your Boat."**
  In this case, this means:
  Remove the toxic pumps from your mouth.

NEXT ACTION:
"Follow the Recipe"…1,2,3…

1. & 2. Dental Revision: Remove and Replace

- *Remove all toxic mercury (silver) amalgam fillings and replace them with non-toxic composite (white) fillings.*

- *Remove root canal teeth. May be replaced with artificial teeth.*

- *Replace any nickel or chrome bridgework with gold or porcelain bridgework.*

I am well aware removing root canal teeth is easier said than done. If you have multiple root canal teeth, this can be done in stages.

3. Practice Oil Pulling 20 minutes every day *to heal gums, avert future infections and to reduce toxic load of microbes in your mouth and in your body.*

Composite Fillings:

The FDA advises that composite fillings are made of a type of acrylic resin and are a common alternative to amalgam fillings. They also inform that composite fillings require a minimum removal of the healthy tooth to apply. As an added bonus, this type of filling may be matched to the particular color or shade of Patient's existing teeth.

"Huggins Applied Healing"...

In 2013, Dr. Blanche Grube joined forces with Dr. Hal Huggins creating the Huggins-Grube Protocol for Biological Dentistry. Dr. Blanche now continues the worldwide education on the need for "Full Dental Revision" to achieve optimal whole body health and healing for every Patient.

IMPORTANT:

Please, DO NOT go to just any Dentist to have your amalgam fillings removed and replaced. You want a Dental Professional who *specializes* in removing and replacing amalgam fillings with *composite (white) fillings.* This is done very carefully by a certain process which protects the Patient from inhaling the mercury vapors of the old filling as it is being removed.

Resources for Safe Removal and Replacement of Amalgam fillings:

- See Holistic Dental Association which is an International Organization of Mercury-Free Dentists. (www.holisticdental.org)

- See Hugginsappliedhealing.com for a list of Dentists that have been trained in the Huggins-Grube Protocol. 866-948-4638

- Other keywords to use in your search:
    Holistic Dentistry
    Mercury-Free Dentistry
    Biological Dentistry
    Environmental Dentistry

Chapter Seven

Reversing Alzheimer's
"The Secret Key"

This Chapter is particularly dear to my heart, as it vividly rekindles memories of my 90-year-old Mother's resurrection from the mental abyss of Alzheimer's Disease. Using very simple *Holistic Methods,* my Mother successfully regained the gift and independence of a clear-thinking mind and reanimated spirit, *in 4 months.* Her entire personality was reactivated and engaging again. For anyone who has a loved one trapped inside their mind or lost within the mental abyss of Dementia or Alzheimer's, I truly hope this Chapter will feel like an answer to your prayers.

What is the Difference between Dementia and Alzheimer's…?

Medical Experts define Dementia as the *Broad Term Bucket* which contains numerous neurological disorders, including Alzheimer's. If you have Alzheimer's, then you have Dementia. However, if you have Dementia, you do not necessarily have Alzheimer's, as there are many other diagnoses in this Bucket, such as: Parkinson's Disease, Lewy Body Dementia, Vascular Dementia, Frontotemporal Dementia, Creutzfeldt-Jakob Disease and Huntington's Disease.

Succinctly put, the term Dementia is generally applied to symptoms caused by *brain cell damage, dysfunction or decline*. These symptoms may include impaired reasoning, reduced thinking skills, declining ability to communicate with others, marked memory decline, personality change or introversion and impaired cognitive or motor skills. One medical opinion is that Alzheimer's is the result of a build-up of *amyloid plaque* in the brain which interferes with the communication between brain cells (neurons*). But it has been proven that the predominant cause is the loss of the brain cells' ability to receive glucose, its food. This causes brain cells to starve, break down and die.*

The unanimous Medical conclusion is that Alzheimer's is a type of Dementia that grows increasingly worse…and is irreversible.

I respectfully disagree.

I have witnessed firsthand the seemingly miraculous reversal of severe Alzheimer's symptoms in my own Mother, in a 4-month period of time. This was achieved by way of a healthy diet, along with the addition of one miracle-producing food. I cannot promise your results will be identical to mine. But you will see in this chapter that *many people have had dramatic reversals or, at the very least, substantial reduction in symptoms, as the result of adding only ONE life-changing food to the Dementia Patients' daily diet; and that is unrefined Coconut Oil.*

What was the Magic Recipe…?

My Mother's daily diet included high protein, 8-10 Tablespoons of unrefined Coconut Oil (Good Fat) and Cellfood drops (Chapter 10). For her, it was the Miracle Recipe.

The Starting Point...

When Mother came to live with me, she exhibited the latter stages of Dementia/Alzheimer's. She weighed only a frail 95 pounds. Her mind, spirit and body were simply shriveled up. At the time, she was 90 years old but behaved like a very young child. I had flown with her from Pennsylvania across the country to where I lived, yet Mother had no idea we were even on a plane. She had no idea how we got to my house or that we spent an entire day traveling. She could not learn which room was hers, nor did she remember what a refrigerator or microwave was. Every night, I had to show her how to brush her teeth. She had no awareness that her husband of 67 years had just died. When viewing photos of her oldest son, then deceased, she looked blankly at the picture and asked who he was. It was heartbreaking to witness. Lastly, she asked me almost every day if we could call her Mother on the phone. Every day, she wanted to speak with her mother, who had been dead for 40 years.

My Mother was underweight, emotionless and seemingly submerged beneath a quicksand of oblivion inside her head.

As I said before, I wasn't having any of it.

The Research...

I quickly embarked on a mission to research all I could on the root cause of Alzheimer's and Dementia. I already had a broad knowledge of holistic healing but never ventured into this particular arena before. I lined up my usual protocol of oxygen-giving circulation-boosting foods and supplements, including Coconut Oil, Essential Oils and Cellfood drops. But the game changer for me was reading the Book by Dr. Mary T. Newport entitled, *Alzheimer's Disease, What If There Was a Cure?* What I found there delighted me beyond belief; but frankly I wasn't all that surprised.

- ***The Key ingredient which Dr. Newport used to successfully reverse her husband's severe Alzheimer's was in fact, Coconut Oil.***

We already learned in Chapter 1 that unrefined Coconut Oil feeds and resuscitates sick and dying cells in the brain and throughout the body. We will dive into Dr. Newport's wonderful Book in a minute. Meanwhile...

I used my collective knowledge of health and wellness to establish a very specific diet in my commitment to resurrect my Mother to again be the loving, engaging person she used to be. Each morning, she had oatmeal with protein powder and 4 Tablespoons of unrefined Coconut Oil. In her tea, I melted 2 Tablespoons of Lecithin granules (Phosphatidylcholine) with another Tablespoon of Coconut Oil. Lunch varied from poached salmon on fresh greens to perhaps a salad to open face tuna melt sandwich, with every single meal having Coconut Oil incorporated into it one way or another. *She was eating at least 8-10 Tablespoons of raw Coconut Oil every day, melted in any food or hot drink.* Somewhere throughout the day I gave her a glass of water with 10 drops of *Cellfood,* a liquid supplement that increases your oxygen and electrolytes while recharging your cells' batteries (*Chapter 10*).

"The Lights Came On..."
(Testimonial from Chapter 1)
After only 2 weeks on Coconut Oil, a wonderful thing happened...*the Lights suddenly came on in Mother's eyes.* One morning she just looked at me and calmly said, *"My*

Mother is dead isn't she?" I replied, *"Yes Mother. She died a very long time ago. You're 90 years old now."* She understood perfectly. She was making the logical conclusion that if she is 90 years old, then her mother can't still be alive. She was achieving clarity. *I was so excited!*

When Mother first arrived at my house, her eyes would just stare blankly, from beneath a thick cloud of detachment. *Now suddenly her eyes had come alive again. She* was looking at me and *truly seeing me with clear eyes which were bright with understanding.* She was engaged. Right before my eyes, my Mother was successfully reconnecting to the outside world again.

I realize it is not prudent for any author to be throwing the word *"Miracle"* around, but as I previously stated, *it sure felt like a Miracle to me.*

Day by day, week by week, Mother's improvements continued. She was steady on her feet again. She was making rational observations and deductions.

Less than 5 months later, my niece was to be married back in Pennsylvania. To attend the wedding meant taking a trip back East with Mother. What a vastly different experience this trip was. Mother was fully engaged in the choosing of her dress and helping me pack for the trip. On the plane, she was chatty and engaging with other passengers. My Mother was back; and I was thrilled and thankful.

At the wedding, Mother looked 20 years younger. Even her complexion was pink again. She went from being a shriveled-up shell of a human being to again being the engaging person we knew her to be. My Aunts and Uncles could not believe the transformation. Well, it *seemed like a Miracle* to them too.

I keep 2 special photos of Mother to hallmark her healing. The first one is from the day she first arrived at my house. It depicted her with that blank stare, sallow skin and empty eyes. The second photo was taken 4 months later at the wedding. The difference between these photos is like night and day. In the latter, Mother's face is glowing with life, and you can clearly see... *the lights are on in her eyes*.

The Brain is Rescued by Good Fat...

In the previous chapters of this book we have identified our body's critical need for *Good Fat*. The daily consumption of *Good Fat is especially* crucial for the health, maintenance and proper function of our brain cells.

- **It is estimated that *the Brain is 50-60% fat in the form of Lipids, Phospholipids and Essential Fatty Acids.***

Similar to electrical wires, *brain cells (neurons)* send and receive a massive amount of electrical impulses per minute. Also like electrical wires, they require a sheath of insulation to cover and protect each neuron. This insulation is referred to as the *Myelin Sheath* which is made up of *mostly fat.* We also learned that every one of our 37 trillion cells are like a water balloon, in that they are surrounded by a soft, *pliable outer wall composed of mostly fat, fatty acids*.

Think about it...

If more than 50% of your brain is made of FAT...then what would be the best way to FEED it...?

It has been proven that Good Fat/Good Fatty Acids are the most crucial requirement for optimal brain health and performance.

273

How to Grow a Healthy Baby Brain
Fun Fact for Pregnant Women…
The brain feeds richly on Good Fat, including *Omega-6 Fatty Acids* found in meat and animal products, and *Omega-3 Fatty Acids*, known as DHA and EPA, found in oily fish.

- *The need for these fats are so critical to the development of a baby's brain that they are stored in the body of the Mother before her baby is born.*

Where are they stored…?

You guessed it. Most of this fat is stored in the Mother's buttocks and hips. (*Well that solves that mystery.*) The remaining amount is stored under the skin throughout the body. This accounts for the fact that *women who are fertile have approximately 2x more body fat as men.* This genius structure on God's part increases the likelihood that, based on these *Good Fat stores*, the baby will be born with a "*large and healthy brain.*" God even put a safeguard in place. The need for *Good Fat* is so essential to the development of a baby's brain that *if a woman's body fat percentage drops too low…she becomes infertile.* (*Pretty amazing, isn't it?*)

During the last 3 months of pregnancy, these stored *Good Fats/Essential Fatty Acids* transfer into the fetus. These fats are not only used to feed the fetus' brain but are also stored in its body. This is the main reason a fetus gains most of its body weight and subcutaneous fat in the third trimester of pregnancy. Since babies are born with underdeveloped brains, their *Good Fat storage enables further brain growth and development, even after birth.*

(*Kier Watson, 2019*)

274

- *The level of healthy Fatty Acids in the Mother's body during pregnancy and in Mother's breast milk post birth, has been directly connected to the child's IQ and learning abilities, as well as their psychological and physiological traits.*

- *Please note:*
  We are NOT referring to any and all fat and being good for the Mother or for the baby. Adipose tissue is stored body fat resulting from consuming more daily calories than are used. This is absolutely NOT the same as stored DHA and EPA which comes from Good, Healthy Fat.

How Does All this Relate to Alzheimer's…?
At every age, Your Brain STILL needs Good Fat to THRIVE.

Causes of Mental Decline…

The Brain is the fattiest organ in your Body. It has been strongly established that the brain needs *Good Fat* to develop and function properly both before and after birth. **This requirement does not go away.** *You recall from Chapter 1 that Good Fats also enable the cell walls (including brain cell walls) to receive food and eject waste.* However, too often our brain's ability to receive crucially needed *Good Fat* is often obstructed by poor diet, ill-health and medication, as follows:

Medication:

The increased use of Cholesterol reducing drugs has been directly related to the increase in cases of Alzheimer's and related neurological disorders. *This may be due to this*

275

medication reducing the Good Fat in the blood along with the Bad Fat.

Poor Diet / Ill Health…

Processed oils and Bad Fats have a profound negative effect on our cell health, especially our brain cell health. *We learned that processed oils, hydrogenated oils and trans fats cause your cell walls to harden. These toxic fats also disable the glucose receptors* on your brain cell walls, *obstructing its ability to receive glucose, its food. Since it can't get into the cells, the glucose just builds up in your blood causing diabetes and other disorders. This is a key indicator that cells are starving, especially brain cells.* Next, the overall health of the Patient falls into a downward spiral and a multitude of symptoms and problems arise. Patient is now needing to be treated for diabetes, neuropathy, impaired vision, heart arrhythmia, edema and related symptoms, *all of which overshadow any awareness that his brain cells are dying.*

In other words, it is highly unlikely that anyone will ever say to you, *"Your blood sugar is very high, so let's treat your starving brain cells."*

Here is the takeaway:

- *Unhealthy processed oils prevent the brain cells from accepting glucose, its food. The glucose then builds up in the blood causing systemic disorders, while the brain cells are starving.*

- *Low-Fat or No-Fat Diets starve brain cells.*

- *MCFA's (Medium Chain Fatty Acids) from unrefined Coconut Oil FEED BRAIN CELLS.*

- *Coconut Oil is converted by the liver into "Ketones," a superfuel that crosses the blood-brain barrier to immediately feed and resuscitate starving brain cells.*

Coconut Oil, Ketones: High Octane Fuel for the Brain…
Once ingested, the liver converts the *Good Fat from* raw Coconut Oil into a cell *Superfuel* called *Ketones*. Once processed in the liver, this *Ketone fuel is then delivered immediately and directly to the brain cells*. We previously learned that *the Good Fat in Coconut Oil does NOT require insulin to get into sick or dying cells. This is why Coconut Oil easily penetrates and feeds starving brain cells, even if their insulin receptors are blocked.*

Short Version…
- **Coconut Oil converts to Ketones in the liver and travels directly to the brain. Ketones do NOT need insulin to enter the cell. It passes easily through the outer and inner walls of sick or starving brain cells to feed and resuscitate them.**

- **It is by this action that symptoms of many neurological disorders are reversed.**

A *high Good Fat Diet* is used worldwide as a proven remedy that successfully treats neurological disorders like epilepsy. Let's now state the obvious: *If Coconut Oil successfully feeds malfunctioning brain cells in an epileptic, then in fact, it is also successfully feeding sick brain cells, period. It should then be no surprise that it can also relieve or substantially improve other neurological disorders.*

277

So Say the Experts...

Feeding the brain high octane Ketone fuel from unrefined Coconut Oil has the ability to relieve or improve neurological impairment, whatever the type, as they all stem from dysfunctional or dying brain cells. Extensive research confirms that the effects of eating good Ketone-producing Fat, like Coconut Oil *"exerts strong neurological effects on social behavior and cognition."*

Tove Hallbrook, Stuart Maudsley, Bronwen Martin, et al. (2012). *Epilepsy Res.*

By using a *High Good Fat Diet*, the recovery of motor skills and cognition were markedly improved in lab animals who had suffered traumatic brain injuries.

Appelberg KS, et al. (2009).

Scientists were able to lessen the accumulation of amyloid plaque in the brain by way of a high *Good Fat Diet.*

Van Da, et al. (2005).

A high Good Fat diet has been proven to reduce brain cell death and seizures.

Tai and Truong. (2007); Tai et al. (2008).

When put on a high Good Fat diet, children demonstrated improved alertness and increased cognitive function as well as better behavior.

Kinsman, et al. (1992); Nordi, et al. (2001); Pulsifer, et al. (2001).

Research asserts that a high Good Fat diet can improve cognitive skills of Alzheimer's patients and patients with Parkinson's Disease.

Reger, et al. (2004); Vanitaille, et al. (2005).

Collectively, the research results from a myriad of differently structured studies confirm that a high *Good Fat* diet offers "*broad range neuroprotective benefits*" when used as a protocol for neurodegenerative disorders.
Tove Hallbrook, Stuart Maudsley, Bronwen Martin, et al. (2012). *Epilepsy Res.*

The above findings were further supported by the Intramural Research Program of the National institute on Aging.

Dr. Mary T. Newport's eye-opening book:
"Alzheimer's Disease, What If There Was a Cure?"...
Dr. Newport is a Pediatric Physician specializing in Neonatology. She was the Founder and Director of the Neonatal Intensive Care Unit in Spring Hill Regional Hospital in Florida. Needless to say, she is a well-educated Physician who was triggered to find an effective solution for her beloved husband's advanced Alzheimer's Disease. Their struggles and final victory over this heart-wrenching disease are beautifully detailed in her book, as follows:

Their Amazing Journey...
Dr. Newport's husband Steve had developed Alzheimer's around 2001. Over the next 7 years, she witnessed his downward spiral which included loss of personality, loss of memory, severely impaired motor skills and communication skills. Much like my own Mother, he had sunken into a mental mire of oblivion. Dr. Newport refused to accept the diagnosis *"there was nothing that could be done"*

to reverse or stop Steve's downward progression. _His Azheimer's was diagnosed as "incurable."_

The Beginning, "free-falling"…

Between 2001 and 2002, Steve's mental and emotional decline had accelerated. He would later refer to this chapter of his life as _"free-falling."_ His memory had greatly diminished and doing math became insurmountable. Lastly, he became severely depressed. By 2003, Dr. Newport took her husband to a Neurologist who performed a _Mini Mental Status Exam_ known as an _MMSE test._ This is a 30-point memory test used to assess the probability of brain dysfunctions including Alzheimer's. This is a simple memory test wherein a healthy normal functioning brain usually achieves a score of 29 or 30. Sadly, Steve scored only a 23. The Neurologist advised it was possibly Alzheimer's but wished to continue to monitor Steve's progression. By 2005, Steve's MMSE score had dropped to 21.

Steve's Symptoms…

Steve systematically hoarded unnecessary items, bunching them up in piles and heaps having no rhyme or reason. He frequently lost his keys and wallet and although he held onto almost everything, he could find nothing when he needed it. His wife realized at some point that Steve could no longer read a map, and that when driving, he would actually turn left when she instructed him to turn right. After ending up in cities that were hours away from his intended destination, she decided that it was unsafe for Steve to continue to drive.

Steve used to be an avid reader. Alarmingly, this fell to the wayside. His wife thought it was because he just lost interest; but Steve later revealed that it was because when

280

he tried to read, the words would jump around on the page. (He later recorded: *The words would become little squares like pixels...and would move rapidly in all different directions.*)

Previously a good cook, Steve eventually abandoned this task after several mishaps with the stove. Also, he had lost 10 pounds. This kind of weight loss was known to indicate a rapid decline in Alzheimer's patients. Also, he began to withdraw from everyday conversations. (He later clarified this was because he couldn't remember what he was saying for longer than 20 seconds.) Lastly, he developed a tremor in his jaw.

When Dr. Newport first met her husband, he was on the wrestling team at school and was always fit and physically strong. By 2007, it was heartbreaking to see that his gait was slow and unsteady with each step needing to be deliberate. He now appeared to be only a shadow of the person she once knew.

For about a year, Steve would walk around with only one shoe on. Steve would go into the silverware drawer looking for a spoon and after much deliberation, he would come away with a knife. This lesson in futility would be repeated up to 4 times before he got it right. His MRI tests explained he had *severe atrophy (shrinking)* of the *hippocampus* part of the brain which controls long-term memory and of the *amygdala,* the part of the brain which governs emotion, learning and memory. In short, *his brain cells were dying off.*

By 2008, Steve had been severely depressed for about 7 years. No medication helped him but in fact only brought side effects to be dealt with. Watching Steve fade away, Dr. Newport faced the dreaded realization that she was slowly losing her husband. Testing in 2008 revealed that Steve had moderate brain shrinkage on one side of his brain, severe shrinkage on the other side and even his prefrontal cortex had shrunken. This is the part of the brain that governs higher thinking and function. *His MMSE score had dropped to an alarming 12. His brain was shrinking because his brain cells were dying of starvation.*

However, there is an ancient axiom that states: *"It is always darkest before dawn."* This was never truer than with what happened next.

An Accidental Discovery...

Unexpectedly one day, Dr. Newport came across new and impressive research findings for the treatment of Alzheimer's Disease. The findings first confirmed that glucose is the primary source of food for brain cells, for all cells. Next, it was confirmed that when neurons (brain cells) are deprived of glucose, they malfunction, producing different consequences with different symptoms depending upon their location in the brain. The results of this are Alzheimer's, Parkinson's, Lou Gehrig's Disease (ALS), Huntington's Disease and other neurological disorders. *Deprived of fuel, the brain cells starve, malfunction and eventually die.* These findings also *attest that in the place of glucose, Ketones (from MCFA's) were proven to be an immediate Superfuel for brain cells. (Ahh but you already learned this in Chapter 1.)*

Dr. Newport found a new drug had just been manufactured for the treatment of Alzheimer's Disease. This drug provided *Ketones bodies* to be used by the brain instead of glucose. Testing showed that the progression of Alzheimer's was slowed down by long-term use of this drug.

The problem was, the drug manufacturer applied for a patent for their drug whose main ingredients were *2 Fatty Acids in MCT Oil which were derived from…Coconut Oil. Talk about taking the long way around the barn!*

Inspired by these findings, Dr. Newport asked herself what any intelligent person would ask:

Where can I find the best natural source of these MCFA's?

She found the answer was: Coconut Oil.

After intensive research, Dr. Newport discovered:

- **<u>MCFA's in Coconut Oil produce Ketones, a powerful Superfuel for the brain.</u>**

- **<u>These Ketones cause circulation in the brain to increase by 39%.</u>**

- **Ketones were proven to cause dramatic improvements in Patients with neurological disorders, such as greatly improved memory, restored personality and cognitive skills, improved motor skills and resumed social interaction.**

She realized this discovery could be life-changing for her and Steve.

Dr. Newport soon discovered that using *MCFA Ketones* instead of glucose to feed brain cells was a known fact. Once available in the bloodstream, *Ketones can bypass the entire glucose/insulin mechanism and pass easily into the sick or dying brain cells to feed them high-octane food to help resuscitate them.*

283

Ketones have the ability to cross the blood/brain barrier and deliver high potency fuel to the brain without opposition. Studies proved they produce a more powerful form of fuel as compared to an equal amount of glucose. With Ketone fuel, ATP production of the cell mitochondria was almost doubled. ATP is an "energy molecule" produced by a healthy cell. Finally, Ketones cause circulation in the brain to increase by 39%. (Hasselbach, 1996)

Coconut Oil is composed of 5 beneficial MCFA's including *Lauric Acid, Caprylic Acid and Capric Acid. MCT Oil is simply a fractionalized version of Coconut Oil. It contains only 2 MCFA's: Caprylic Acid (75%) and Capric Acid (25%). Specifically, it is the Caprylic Acid (C:8) that has the most dramatic effect on the brain.* As a Pediatrician, Dr. Newport clearly recalled her medical training included the widespread use of MCT Oil (Fractionalized Coconut Oil) to nourish premature babies because it is so easily absorbed by their underdeveloped digestive systems. It also supports their brain development and immune system. Because of these unique benefits, MCT Oil was a standard ingredient in almost all infant formulas, and many Neonatal Care Units still use this today. (Tantibhehlyangkul, 1975)

Since Coconut Oil is 60% MCFA's, Dr. Newport concluded that *just 2 Tablespoons of Coconut Oil would be equal to 20 grams of MCT Oil,* the same dosage that was in the new Alzheimer's drug. The question was: *Could a simple food like raw Coconut Oil resuscitate brain cells enough to bring her husband back from his 8-year downward spiral…?*

The Miraculous Month of May…

284

May 20, 2008, Screening #1:

Unfortunately, after all these exciting discoveries, Dr. Newport didn't have time to give Steve any Coconut Oil before bringing him for his MMSE test on this particular day. Sadly, even after being reminded many times, he still couldn't remember the word Spring or even what day or what month it was. *Although they "studied" for his test, he only scored a very low 14 out of 30.*

The Clock:

On this same appointment, Steve's Neurologist asked him to draw a clock. This task was a type of informal test which specifically indicated the level of Alzheimer's. When asked to do so, Steve produced an odd-looking drawing having three tiny unrelated circles the size of raisins located in random sections of the paper, along with 4 scattered numbers. It seemed like the drawing of a very small child. *The Doctor assessed that Steve's mental decline was now severe.*

May 21, 2008, Screening #2 / Day 1 of Coconut Oil:

The next day, Dr. Newport was prepared. She arose early enough to make a nice bowl of hot oatmeal for Steve, *adding just 2 Tablespoons of Coconut Oil to it.* That would be the equivalent of 20 grams of MCT Oil. Incredibly, on this 2nd MMSE test, *Steve scored an 18. This was 4 points higher than the day before! The Neurologist considered this to be a drastic improvement.*

- *The only explanation was the Coconut Oil.*

Could this really be happening? Was it really this simple all along?

Dr. Newport held her breath and continued the Coconut Oil treatment for her husband, adding it faithfully to his oatmeal every morning.

Day 3 on Coconut Oil:

Prior to eating Coconut Oil, Steve would wander into the kitchen as if in a fog. Hardly speaking at all, he fumbled to find his utensils and would eventually find the table, finally sitting down and eating very slowly.

However, after *only three days* of being on Coconut Oil, Dr. Newport recorded that Steve came into the kitchen *"alert, smiling, talkative and happy!"* Suddenly it was no longer a problem to locate his utensils and he even got himself a glass of water.

Day 5 on Coconut Oil:

Steve attested that suddenly *"he felt as if a light had switched on, the fog had lifted, and his life had changed for the better."* Dr. Newport advises that by Day 5, *"Steve and I looked at each other and agreed our life had changed."*
(Newport, 2011)

May 26, 2008:

Dr. Newport records she is now giving Steve Coconut Oil multiple times a day. Steve has been *"alert and happy"* *every day so far.* He is remembering dreams and even events from first grade. This day he cleaned the pool, vacuumed 2 rooms of the house then went out to do gardening.

Dr. Newport advises she now puts Coconut Oil in her husband's Oatmeal, in smoothies, on his baked potato and she is even using it to cook with. Steve likes the flavor.

May 28, 2008:

Every day so far, Steve appears very happy and alert. He now easily knows what day, month and season it is. Yet only 7 days ago, he couldn't remember any of these things, even after being repeatedly coached.

May 29, 2008:

Steve continues to be alert and active. He took apart the pool pump and cleaned it, reassembling all the small parts almost perfectly. He appears more "normal" each day. Still sometimes struggles to find correct words.

May 30, 2008:

Steve still appears happy, alert and "normal." He even went to get the newspaper. For the first time in many years, he read a few pages of a magazine. He is able to empty and reload the dishwasher. By evening, he is still very alert. They are having good conversations.

June 1, 2008:

Steve is getting up early, alert and talkative. We now discuss many things from politics to Coconut Oil. His gait is visibly improving.

June 3, 2008 / Day 14 on Coconut Oil / Clock #2:

Steve continues to awake alert and enthused for the day. Today, he was asked to draw Clock #2. What a huge improvement it was from just 2 weeks ago! This drawing actually looked very much like a clock, having a big circle containing lines radiating from the center of the circle to the ends and he even numbered them from 1 through 12. The numbers were a wee bit messy and not all the same size but they were inserted in perfect order 1 through 12.

- *This drawing of Clock #2 clearly reflected the amazing level of healing the Coconut Oil had on Steve's brain cells, in just 2 short weeks.*

June 26 / Day 37 on Coconut Oil / Clock #3:

Steve drew clock #3. His placement of numbers on this clock were much better and the concentric spokes coming out of the center of the clock were much more even, like a bicycle wheel. His tremors have diminished, and his gait is almost normal.

During her research, Dr. Newport happened upon a world-renowned Ketone Expert named Richard L. Veech, M.D. a Biochemist and Metabolic Specialist and in the National Institute of Health in Bethesda Maryland. One of his many successful studies was recorded in a document called "*Review: The Therapeutic Implications of Ketone Bodies published in Prostaglandins and Essential Fatty Acids.*"
(Veech, 2004)

- *Consistent with previous findings, Dr. Veech asserted that Ketones from MCFA's can be successfully used to feed brain cells (neurons) in patients with Alzheimer's and Parkinson's Disease as these patients are unable to utilize glucose for brain fuel.*
Steve was already living proof of this.

Dr. Newport contacted Dr. Veech who asserted that Coconut Oil would provide the proper MCFA's to make the needed Ketones to feed the brain cells of patients with neurological disorders. He said some patients try to use MCT Oil, but the MCT Oil can cause diarrhea. Lastly, Dr. Veech basically advised that *it appeared that the medical and political arena were not informed enough to recognize the profound effect that Ketones (MCFA's) have on disease.*

Letter to Supreme Court Justice…

Dr. Newport was eager to spread the word about this simple but amazing treatment for Alzheimer's and other neurodegenerative diseases. She wrote a detailed letter to Supreme Court Justice, Sandra O'Connor, who was also a member of the Alzheimer's Study Group (ASG). Her letter revealed the following:

"Science has asserted that the brain cells of Alzheimer's, Parkinson's and Huntington's Disease patients are not able to receive Glucose which causes them to malfunction and die. It has been further proven that Ketones from MCFA's from Coconut Oil and MCT Oil have been proven to successfully feed and resuscitate these neurons (brain cells).

The Fatty Acids from Coconut Oil are not processed like any other fats. They are not stored by the body like other fats. These MCFA's are taken up by the liver where they are converted into Ketones and pass readily into the brain. Once this occurs, blood flow to the brain increases by 39%. Research confirms that Coconut Oil does not raise cholesterol; but in fact lowers bad cholesterol.

Cultures that use Coconut Oil as a daily staple have a much lower incidence of degenerative and cardiovascular disease. Coconut Oil is vastly healthier and more health-giving fat than processed and hydrogenated vegetable oils that have infected the western diet." (Newport, 2011)

In her letter, Dr. Newport also relayed the great success she had with her husband in only two weeks of being on Coconut Oil: His gait is almost normal, he is conversant, his personality and sense of humor has been restored. He is alert and engaged again. She went on to say she was alarmed and disappointed that a drug company would try to patent a "new Alzheimer's drug" whose *miracle ingredient was simply MCFA's derived from Coconut Oil...an over the counter health food.*

The Family Visit...

After only 30 days on Coconut Oil, Dr. Newport and her husband Steve went on a family visit. The family recalled that only a year ago, Steve was introverted and non-communicative. He had no sense of humor or interest in his family or in his surroundings. They remembered that he didn't even know their names. However, on this visit a year later, Steve was alert and engaged. He greeted everyone by name, had lively conversations and even made jokes like the old Steve would do. The family agreed that the change in him was no less than "remarkable."

Day 65 on Coconut Oil:

Steve scored a 20 on his MMSE test. That's 2 points higher than the last test and 6 points higher than the first one.

Dr. Newport had bloodwork done on Steve to measure the difference in his Ketone levels when taking Coconut Oil and again after taking MCT Oil. *The results showed that the Coconut Oil caused Steve's plasma Ketones to stay level much longer than did the MCT Oil*, which peaked sooner but then dropped much sooner. Also, only the MCT Oil sometimes caused vomiting or diarrhea, whereas the *Coconut Oil did not.*

Month 4 on Coconut Oil:

Dr. Newport recorded the following improvements for Steve after taking Coconut Oil for 4 months:

- *Facial tremors disappeared*
- *Increased alertness and happiness*
- *Increased ability to have in-depth conversations*
- *Increased libido*
- *No longer distracted off tasks*
- *Compete recognition of family members*
- *Increased desire to exercise and learn*
- *Ability to read again*
- *All instances of words "jumping around on the page" had vanished*
- *Walking gait is normal*
- *Depression gone*
- *He can run*

April 2009 / One Year on Coconut Oil:

Previously, Steve's MRI tests had shown alarming brain shrinkage occurring between 2004 and 2008. Dr. Newport expected there would still be some signs of additional shrinkage on this year's MRI as well. *However, she was amazed to learn that there was NO more brain shrinkage whatsoever since the last MRI a year ago. This was further confirmation that the Ketones from Coconut Oil were keeping her husband's brain cells alive.*

A Day Without Coconut Oil...

One day while traveling, Steve went without his Coconut Oil. His tremors returned. He became shaky and confused. He began fumbling with his utensils.

His wife realized he hadn't had any Coconut Oil that day. She proceeded to give him a dose of Coconut Oil. In only 30 minutes, Seve's tremors ceased and he became stable and clear minded again.

Dr. Newport proceeded to write an article on the extraordinary progress her husband had made while taking Coconut Oil. Dr. Bruce Fife, author of *The Coconut Oil Miracle* published Dr. Newport's amazing success story in his newsletter, *Healthy Ways.* Steve's great success with Coconut Oil was also published in the *St. Petersburg Times* in a story entitled *"Sketches in Progress"* by Eve Hosley-Moore.

2011 / 3 years on Coconut Oil:
Dr. Newport happily reports that Steve has retained all achieved improvements.
Steve continues to take 3 Tablespoons of Coconut Oil (sometimes mixed with MCT Oil) at each meal plus another 2 Tablespoons before bed. That is 11 Tablespoons per day.
- *Despite eating all this Good Fat every day, Steve had lost 10 pounds.*
- *Also, his triglycerides had dropped and his Good Cholesterol had tripled.*

Dr. Newport was haunted by the belief that Ketones from Coconut Oil could be a true cure for Alzheimer's and other neurodegenerative diseases. At the very least, it could reverse or improve neural degeneration by resuscitating starved and dying brain cells. She and Steve attended the National Alzheimer's Association and Conference. Steve gave a sad synopsis of the event observing that it just seemed like a group of people wrestling for funding. He ended by stating to his wife, *"You had the cure in your hand, and they ignored you."*

Finally, in the Newsletter *Health and Healing,* an article called *"A Breakthrough in Alzheimer's Disease"* was published in October 2009 by Dr. Julian Whitaker, Founder of the world famous Whitaker Wellness Institute. This story celebrated Dr. Newport and her husband's journey through their successful reversal of Alzheimer's Disease.

Johns Hopkins Researchers Confirm
Successful Treatment of Neurological Disorders with Good Fats...

In 2010, Dr. Newport and Steve attended an International Symposium on Dietary Intervention for Epilepsy and other Neurological Disorders. A supporter of this Conference was Dr. Dominic D'Agostino Ph.D., who successfully treated a Patient with severe treatment-resistant seizures. Remarkably, the Patient's seizures were completely eliminated by way of a High Good Fat Diet (Ketone producing Fats).

A *Ketogenic Diet is one that is* low in Carbohydrates and *very high in "Good Fats" like raw Coconut Oil.* At this Global Symposium were the cream of the crop experts from Johns Hopkins School of Medicine who researched Ketogenic Foods for the successful treatment of Neurological disorders. This included Pediatric Neurologists Eric Kossoff M.D., Adam Hartman M.D., and Eileen Vinings M.D.

Their Research results unanimously confirmed:

- *Even relatively low blood levels of Ketones from Good Fat produced substantial improvements in Neurological Disorders.*

- *Patients with severe seizures achieved great reduction or complete relief from seizures when eating Ketone producing Fats.*

Ketones Shrink Cancer Cells and Tumors....

Thomas Seyfried, Ph.D., a Professor of Biology at the University of Illinois, was one of the renowned researchers who specialized in the use of Ketone-Producing Fats to treat brain cancer. His presentation attested his discovery that certain types of brain cancer, such as *glioblastoma, can shrink by up to 80%* as a result of being on a Ketone-producing, high Good Fat diet. The additional benefit of this dietary treatment is that once the tumors shrink, then it becomes safe for it to be surgically removed with much less risk to the Patient.

However, his most amazing revelation was that he found that cancer cells live on glucose...NOT Ketones.

- **By feeding the body Ketones for fuel instead of glucose, Cancer cells starve while healthy cells thrive.**

Dr. Siegfried et al performed a case study on a 65-year-old Patient whose tumor shrunk so small that it was no longer detectable on a PET scan or an MRI. This amazing remission resulted from his Patient being on a diet high in Ketone-Producing Good Fats for only 2 months.
(Zuccoli, 2010)

Alzheimer's: Brain Cell Death, BrainShrinkage (Atrophy)...

Alzheimer's is described as having loss of brain cells and loss of proper cell function in various parts of the brain.

This includes the temporal, parietal and frontal lobes, prefrontal cortex, the entorhinal cortex and hippocampus. In latter stages, the cerebral cortex is damaged. This area governs language, social behavior and reasoning. *The root cause being the brain cells' inability to receive glucose, their life-sustaining food. They then malfunction and eventually die off. This is brain cell "atrophy" or shrinkage. This is basically brain cell death.*

It is still generally believed that the mechanism of Alzheimer's Disease remains *"unknown and irreversible."*

…Yet again, I respectfully disagree.

Testimonials…
Successful Treatment of Alzheimer's with Coconut Oil

My Mother, a 90-Year-Old Woman with Dementia / Alzheimer's…
(Testimony from Chapter 1)

My Mother came to live with me in January, 2014. Although we spent all day traveling, she had no awareness that we were even on a plane. At my house, she had no idea where she was or how she got there. She did not recognize a refrigerator or a microwave. She did not care about her appearance. Each night I had to show her how to brush her teeth. She repeated questions and could not process the answers. She was not aware that her husband and oldest son were dead. Lastly, at 90 years old, she kept asking me to call her Mother, who had been dead for 40 years. My Mother was underweight, frail and emotionless. Her skin was dull, and her eyes were distant and cloudy, reflecting the thick mental fog that she was living behind.

I started her immediately on a *High Protein/High Good Fat Diet including unrefined Coconut Oil.* Reading Dr. Mary Newport's Book, *Alzheimer's Disease, What if There was a Cure?* further confirmed to me that the MCFA's in Coconut Oil feed and *resuscitate sick and dying brain cells.* I then increased Mother's Coconut Oil dosage to 8-10 Tablespoons per day. I put it in her food, in her tea, in her smoothies, on her vegetables and even on her raisin toast. Mother improved rapidly from there.

The Lights came on in Her Eyes...

After just a few short weeks on Coconut Oil, Mother walked up to me one day being calm and clear minded. She remembered her mother was dead. She realized where she was. Suddenly she understood almost everything. I was both stunned and thrilled.

My Mother's improvements continued and were amazing. Mother was looking at me and truly seeing me with clear eyes which were bright with understanding. She was engaged. Right before my eyes, my Mother was successfully reconnecting to the outside world again. As the weeks passed by, Mother's improvements mounted. She was making rational observations and decisions. As I have previously stated...*it sure felt like a Miracle to me.*

After 4 months on Coconut Oil...

My Niece was getting married back in Pennsylvania. To attend the wedding meant taking a flight back East with Mother. What a vastly different experience this trip was! She was chatty and engaging with other passengers on the plane, just like the old version of herself would be. My Mother was back; and I was thrilled and thankful.

At the wedding, Mother looked 20 years younger. Even her complexion was pink again. She went from being a shriveled-up shell of a human being to again being the charming person we all knew her to be. My Aunts and Uncles could not believe the transformation. *It seemed like a Miracle to them too.*

As I previously shared, I keep 2 special photos of Mother to hallmark her healing. The first one is from the day she first arrived at my house. It depicts her with that blank stare, sallow skin and those cloudy, empty eyes. The second photo was taken 4 months later at the wedding. The difference between these photos is like night and day. In the latter photo, Mother's skin is pink, her face is glowing with life, and you can clearly see…*the lights are on in her eyes.*

Alzheimer's Disease, What If There Was a Cure ? (2011)

In her Book, Dr. Mary Newport records 60 healing Testimonials from Caregivers of Dementia Patients. She brought those reports to the International Symposium on Dietary Intervention for Epilepsy and other Neurological Disorders. The following amazing healings are derived from some of those testimonials, as follows:

77-Year-Old Man with Alzheimer's

After only 2 weeks of being on Coconut Oil, Patient's wife affirms she is delighted to see a huge difference in her husband. He's feeding their pets again, properly setting the table for his meals, and getting his own breakfast cereal. She can hardly believe this dramatic change is from a simple thing like Coconut oil.

She concludes by saying, "To me, his improvement is a Miracle."

83-Year-Old Woman with Dementia

This Patient's daughter described that her Mother would *"just sit in a chair all day like a vegetable."* Her Mother

297

would not engage with anyone and didn't recognize family members or even her husband. She was also very unsteady on her feet.

After 7 weeks on Coconut Oil, her Mother became increasingly more coherent and "the dead look behind her eyes was clearing." She began walking better as well as remembering and recognizing people much better. The most profound change was that one day she said she wanted to read the newspaper! (Daughter advised her Dad almost passed out.) Her Daughter declares "the transformation (in her Mother) is truly a Miracle."

After 6 months on Coconut Oil, Patient's Daughter advises her mother is now knitting again. Six months ago she couldn't even remember what the needles were used for.

After 1 Year on Coconut Oil, Patient is doing extremely well on 8 Tablespoons of Coconut Oil and MCT Oil a day. Her daughter is still in disbelief as she watches her mother actually having real conversations with her Father, being alert, happy and playing with her great-grandchildren again.

Daughter attests that it is hard to believe that only a year ago, her Mother was combative, refused to eat, soiled herself and didn't remember who anyone was. What a difference now! She thanks Dr. Newport for all her diligent work in sharing this simple yet remarkable Coconut Oil treatment.

80-Year-Old Woman with Dementia

After reading Dr. Newport's Article, this Caregiver started giving her Mother Coconut Oil every day. In only 4 weeks, Caregiver affirms she *"sees marked improvement in her Mother's cognition and function."*

78-Year-Old Man with Dementia / Frontal Lobe

Patient's wife confirms her husband has improved significantly with the Coconut Oil. His speaking is now improved, and he is remembering words much better.

After 5 Months, *Patient has been taking 3 teaspoons of Coconut Oil + 4 teaspoons of MCT Oil 3x a day. Before taking the Coconut Oil and MCT Oil he would demonstrate bizarre behavior, like melting a CD in the toaster, and starting fires by putting dish towels in the microwave. His wife attests she is relieved and thankful that "his behavior has dramatically improved since he has been on the Oils."*

90-Year-Old Woman with Dementia

Caregiver's Mother only scored an 18 out of 30 on her MMSE/Mental assessment test. After starting a daily regimen of Coconut Oil and MCT Oil, her Mother exhibited much more energy. She was more coherent and much happier than before. Daughter affirms, *when retested, her Mother scored a 26 out of 30, that is 8 points higher on her Mental assessment test!*

The daughter confirmed that her Mother is now attending parties, church and exercise classes, which she hasn't done in 10 years.

56-Year-Old Man with Dementia…

After only a few weeks of taking Coconut Oil and MCT Oil, Patient's wife attests that she is witnessing more improvement in him each day. She is amazed that sometimes her husband seems so normal now that she "forgets he has any problem at all."

After 2 months on Coconut Oil and MCT Oil, *unexpected and* <u>fabulous news came with Patient's Blood</u> <u>Test results. Patient's wife attests that his Cholesterol</u>

DROPPED from 140 to 120; his Triglycerides DROPPED from 100 to 58 (almost half); and his LDL's (Bad Cholesterol) DROPPED from 70 to 54.

Eating Good Healthy Fat 3x a day caused this Patient to have the best blood test results he has seen in 4 years.

Wife advises that improvements for her husband continue each month. He is conversant, helping around the house, grilling food and generally participating in life again. He even remembers to relay a message if someone calls while she's out.

A profound event was when her husband asked to go to the camera store. Once there, he was able to clearly articulate what kind of camera he needed and exactly what he wanted to do with it. *Wife declares she was totally shocked.*

83-Year-Old Man with Dementia

Caregiver attests she found immediate relief of her husband's symptoms once he started taking Coconut Oil. Unfortunately, naysayers advised her to stop the treatment, warning her that it may raise her husband's cholesterol (although the exact opposite is true). But when she stopped the Coconut Oil, she was alarmed to see that her husband "started going backwards." She then resumed giving him the Coconut Oil each day with only good results and no negative side effects to his cholesterol. Seeing is believing.

87-Year-Old Man with Vascular Dementia

Patient's Daughter attests that before taking Coconut Oil, her Dad would lay in bed all day and have disturbing episodes at night. He was not talking and did not recognize family members.

After Only 5 Days on Coconut Oil, Daughter confirms her Dad is becoming more like himself every day, getting out of bed himself, suddenly recognizing people and engaging them in conversation. After only 5 days, her Dad is now out of bed and walking around seemingly "recognizing everything" and accomplishing things he hasn't done in a long while. Daughter advises her Mom "calls it a Miracle."

91-Year-Old Woman with Alzheimer's Disease

Patient's Daughter attests she is convinced that the Coconut Oil has helped her Mother. Prior to taking it each day, her Mother would attempt to write grocery lists which became increasingly more and more illegible. After taking the Coconut Oil, the lists suddenly became *"astoundingly more readable,"* being properly written along lines of the paper with only a few misspellings. Also, her Mother was now easily engaging in phone conversations whereas before, she couldn't even hold the phone to her ear.

62-Year-Old Man with Early Onset Alzheimer's

After reading Dr. Newport's Blog about Coconut Oil, Patient's wife began giving her husband 3-4 teaspoons of Coconut Oil and MCT Oil 3x a day. After 6 weeks, she found that her husband was able to read again and also retain what he read. He became more engaging and sociable, and is even able to write lecture notes into his ledger. He was less depressed and his tremors have improved. For the first time in a year, he wrote some emails and also asked his wife to put some money into his wallet.

63-Year-Old Man with Early onset Alzheimer's

Patient's Daughter advises her Dad had begun slipping into the Alzheimer's quicksand since 2008. His family feared they were losing him. After reading Dr. Newport's Article, Patient started taking just ONE Tablespoon of Coconut Oil a day. After only 3 weeks, Daughter reports that *her Dad is now more focused, converses more easily and just seems "sharper."* She claims, *"It's amazing."*

The Daughter further confirms that her entire family is now taking Coconut Oil every day.

57-Year-Old Woman with Early Onset Alzheimer's

Patient's husband advised that his beloved wife started having Alzheimer's symptoms in 2007. In 2010, *her Neurologist advised there was <u>no cure</u>*. Two days later, her husband found Dr. Newport's website about the successful use of Coconut Oil. *Patient began taking 2 Tablespoons 3x a day. Improvement in his wife was visible after only 2 weeks. Her husband then added MCT Oil 3x a day. Patient became much improved.*

Her Husband attests that before taking Coconut Oil, his wife had become aggressive. She had difficulty dressing, putting her clothes on inside out if at all, and putting her shoes on the wrong foot. She no longer cared about her appearance and had abandoned all interest in even combing her hair. She had no interest in their Grandchildren, not really remembering who they were. She was unable to read a clock. She felt lost whenever they went out and didn't know where she was.

Her husband confirms that after several weeks of taking the Coconut Oil and MCT Oil, his wife's personality has changed completely "as if a switch has been flicked." She is now dressing herself and is even watching her favorite TV programs again. She is once again taking great care of her appearance. She now spends hours playing with her grandchildren. She can now tell what time it is and she is very comfortable when going out shopping.

The Patient's children were shocked at the change in their Mother. Now they are all taking Coconut Oil.

Other Neurological Disorders Successfully Treated with Coconut Oil:
Woman in Coma after Car Accident

This Patient's Mother advised that her Daughter suffered severe brain trauma as a result of a car accident. She had been in a "vegetative state" for a month. After being moved to a Rehabilitation center, *the Patient was given MCT Oil 3x a day. Incredibly, just a few days later, she awoke from her coma and was deemed well enough to begin Physical Therapy. Her Doctor advised he expected the Patient to make a full recovery.*

62-Year-Old Woman with Leaning Syndrome and Alzheimer's

Patient had severe Leaning Syndrome, having her body leaning profoundly to the left. When eating, she would have to lay her head on the person's shoulder sitting to her left. Her balance was very poor and about 98% of her speech was too garbled to understand. Patient had lost all living skills as well as her long and short-term memory. Her eyes were foggy and glazed over. Each month she contracted a cold accompanied by cold sores (herpes virus). Lastly, she endured dizziness, fainting spells and cold sweats.

On Day 1 *of taking Coconut Oil, the Caretaker confirmed Patient's eyes appeared "clear and alert." Improvements appeared each week.*

303

- **After 5 months** on Coconut Oil and MCT Oil, the Caregiver records that <u>Patient's Leaning Syndrome is completely gone</u>.
  (& there's that "Miracle" word raising its hand again!)

Caregiver reported that astonishingly, the Patient is now able to walk straight with much better balance. Her speech is 65% coherent. She can now perform some daily tasks without prompting. Her short-term memory is improved, she remembers her name and date of birth. She now has the ability to remember other people's names and to learn new names. Since starting the Coconut/ MCT Oils, Patient has had only 1 cold and 1 cold sore; this happened as a result of lowering the Coconut Oil dosage. The Patient has had only 1 episode of dizziness/fainting in 5 months. Lastly, <u>her cholesterol has dropped</u>.

72-Year-Old Man with Parkinson's Disease

After suffering Parkinson's Disease for 10 years, this Patient has had remarkable success with Coconut Oil, taking about 6 grams of it every day. His Caregiver reports he has had a *substantial reduction in tremors, he is eating well and even works out 4 days a week. Patient has improvement in bowel movements, agility and memory. When they run out of Coconut Oil, there is a marked decline in Patient's mental clarity and motor function.*

Woman with Glaucoma

This Patient had intelligently concluded that since Coconut Oil helps feed and resuscitate brain cells, then it must have a benefit for her Glaucoma. Her assumption was based upon the fact that Glaucoma is a neurodegenerative disorder and that the retinal (eye) neurons are directly connected to the neurons in the brain. She began taking only 3 Tablespoons of Coconut Oil a day. By the second night, she was seeing her computer screen with increased ease and clarity, even discerning colors of blue and pink she had never seen there before. One day, the toolbar looked gray to her. She took a Tablespoon of Coconut Oil and *within about 30 minutes*, she was able to discern the toolbar was the color pink again.

Patient attests she then increased her dosage of coconut Oil to 8 Tablespoons per day. She is now able to see better and drive at night with increased depth perception. She states she is excited that the improvements in her vision are dramatic and ongoing.

16-year-old Boy with Seizures

This Mother reported that her son used to suffer regular daily seizures including a Grand Mal seizure every night. Only a few days after starting him on Coconut Oil he skipped a day of having any seizures including the evening Grand Mal. More importantly, her son began to read again and was able to comprehend an entire book, which he was unable to do before taking Coconut Oil. One day, her son had 2 meals cooked in Coconut Oil, 2 Tablespoons plus 6 capsules of it. He went outside in the heat of the day, running around and playing frisbee without having a seizure. He was chatty alert and helping around the house. He has gone 3 days without a single Grand Mal seizure. His Mother reports, *"Yesterday we skipped his dose of Coconut Oil, and his Grand Mal came back."*

Huntington's Disease

Patient's Wife reported that her husband's family has

a history of Huntington's Disease and that her husband had recently developed symptoms. *She started him on Coconut Oil and MCT Oil at each meal which "kept his symptoms at bay." His Wife confirmed that if she lessened his dosage, then his random, unintentional movements and unsteady gait would return.*

62-Year-Old Man with ALS / FALS (Familial Amyotrophic Lateral Sclerosis)

After suffering from a major muscle loss in his leg, this Patient was diagnosed with ALS/FALS 3 years ago. After watching videos from Dr. Newport about her Coconut Oil success, he began taking it. Patient reports he started with 2 Tablespoons a day and increased it to *8 Tablespoons a day.* In less than a year, he has had very positive results. Patient reports that *incredibly, he has gained some muscle mass in his upper right leg. Prior to taking the Coconut Oil, he could feel nothing but bone when he reached behind his leg, whereas now he feels muscle. He further confirmed that his leg now feels "more awake and like a part of him again."* He admits it is still not perfect, but it is substantially better. Lastly, *Patient confirms despite taking 8 Tablespoons of Coconut Oil a day, his blood tests came back good with all things normal including his cholesterol.*

47-Year-Old Man with Parkinson's Disease (Testimony also in Chapter 1)

One of the students in my Health and Wellness Class had a husband suffering from Parkinson's Disease. This was a relatively young man who was now stumbling and falling when he walked, and having great difficulty getting up and down the stairs. This impairment was growing worse each

306

week. It was a huge burden and worry for his family. They feared without a Miracle he would end up in a wheelchair.

Parkinson's Disease is a degenerative disorder of the brain and central nervous system resulting in motor skills degeneration. It has been found to be caused by cell death in the midbrain. Knowing how well Coconut Oil worked to resuscitate my Mother's brain cells, I instructed my student to throw out every other kind of oil in their kitchen and use only unrefined Coconut Oil for all cooking, for everything. I also directed that her husband take 6-8 Tablespoons of unrefined Coconut Oil every day, mixed into his smoothies and hot food or drinks. I also recommended a High Protein Diet.

His improvements increased every week. In a matter of weeks, he was dramatically better. In less than 6 weeks, he had regained his balance, he was exercising again, and he even went back to work. His brain cells were resuscitated by eating Coconut Oil every day. The removal of bad fat and addition of Coconut Oil had very likely prevented this man from ending up in a wheelchair.

A simple choice, a simple food, radically changed this man's health and his life.

To Sum It All Up…

A multitude of renowned Institutions and Medical Experts have confirmed that Neurological Disorders are caused by starving brain cells, which cannot receive glucose, its food. These brain cells then weaken, malfunction and die, causing a host of neurological disorders and diseases. It has been further proven that Ketones are Superfuel for brain cells and are derived from Good Fat (MCFA's). Unrefined Coconut Oil is the highest in these brain-feeding MCFA's, with MCT Oil coming in second.

- Ketones from Coconut Oil do NOT require insulin to enter sick or dying brain cells. *Unrefined Coconut Oil have been proven to be the most powerful Ketone-producing fat, which easily and successfully feeds and resuscitates sick and dying brain cells.*

  - *The Fatty Acids from Coconut Oil are not processed like any other fats. They are not stored by the body like other fats.*

  - *MCFA's from Coconut Oil are taken up by the liver where they are converted into ketones and pass readily into the brain. This causes blood flow to the brain to increase by 39%.*

  - *All research confirms that Coconut Oil does NOT raise cholesterol; but in fact lowers triglycerides and "bad" cholesterol.*

  - *Ketones from Coconut Oil MCFA's can be successfully used to feed brain cells (neurons) in patients with Alzheimer's and Parkinson's Disease, as these patients are unable to utilize glucose for brain fuel. (Veech, 2004)*

The added benefit of eating Coconut Oil is that Native Cultures who use it as a daily staple have a much lower incidence of degenerative and cardiovascular disease. Coconut Oil is vastly healthier and more health-giving fat than the many processed oils which have infected the western diet. Remember, it is the processed oils, hydrogenated oils and trans-fat (Bad Fats) which induce cell shutdown in the first place.

Science has asserted that the brain cells of Alzheimer's, Parkinson's and Huntington's Disease patients are not able to receive glucose which causes them to starve, malfunction and die. It has been further proven that Ketones from MCFA's from Coconut Oil and MCT Oil have been proven to successfully feed and resuscitate these brain cells. (Newport, 2011)

After reversing the symptoms of her husband's "severe and incurable" Alzheimer's, Dr. Mary Newport heralds the belief that Ketones from Coconut Oil and MCT Oil could be a true cure for Alzheimer's and other neurodegenerative diseases. Proven by Science and confirmed by a wide spectrum of stunning Testimonials, Coconut Oil has demonstrated its extraordinary ability to halt, reverse or dramatically improve neural degeneration by resuscitating starving and dying brain cells.

The Secret Key to unlocking Alzheimer's Disease is Unrefined Coconut Oil.

Chapter Eight

"The Budwig Protocol"
Alternative Cancer Treatment

I'll wager that you will find the information in this chapter to be the hardest to believe.

Firstly, at this point in your learning journey I hope you are convinced that *the most powerful of all healing methods are actually the simplest.* Secondly, you are here *to discover proven, uncommon, unknown natural healing methods. So, open your mind to receive*; because the protocol in this chapter is both simple yet amazing, and well, someone much smarter than both of us has proven it to be true.

Dr. Johanna Budwig was born in Germany 1908. She is highly esteemed as one of the foremost experts in Cancer Research, Biochemistry and Pharmacology in the world. In addition to being a Blood Specialist, she is considered one of the world's leading authorities on Fats and Oils (Lipids). Proving what profound effects different kinds of fats/oils have on the human body, as well as confirming the cause and successful treatment of Cancer was her life's work.

For her profound discoveries, <u>Dr. Budwig was nominated for a Nobel Prize…7 times</u>.

(Please read that again.)

The Science…

We previously discussed how each one of our 37 trillion cells is like a tiny water balloon, being surrounded by a soft pliable outer wall (cell membrane) made of fat. Our cell walls are exceedingly thin,10-80 nm (nanometers) depending on what type of cell it is. This microscopically thin cell wall is the only thing standing between the health of the cell and the outside environment. A healthy cell wall is permeable, that is, it allows things to pass into and out of it. By this mechanism, a cell takes in nutrients and oxygen and ejects waste. *A healthy cell repairs and reproduces itself.* These crucial minute by minute cell functions ensure the life and health of our entire body. Individual cell health governs the very core of our overall longevity and vitality. Any interference with the cell's life-giving actions triggers sickness in the cell, and in the body overall.

By now you have learned that when a healthy cell is deprived of oxygen and nutrients it begins to malfunction. Its outer wall becomes hard and impermeable (yes like an M&M candy). So, it can no longer accept food or oxygen; it can no longer eject waste and toxins. It can no longer reproduce. The cell then becomes a breeding nest for infection and disease, including cancer.

Food, oxygen, nutrients, vitamins, minerals, cannot enter a diseased cell. If left untreated, sickness accelerates in the cells, expanding into the organs triggering disorders and disease throughout the body.

The Culprit…
Dr. Budwig confirmed in 1952 that Processed Oils and Fats are a Primary cause of Cellular Breakdown, Disease and Cancer.

- *Processed oils and fats hardened the cell walls and shut down their insulin receptors. No food gets in; no oxygen gets in; no toxins get out. The cell festers in its own waste, breeding sickness and disease, including cancer.*

- *Processed oils and fats kill the cell's electrical charge, making it a "dead battery."*
The cell cannot reproduce. Tumors develop.

Our Bodies are Electric…

We learned in Chapter 2 (*Essential Oils*) that our bodies are *electric*. Dr. Budwig knew this 70 years ago. She confirmed that the center of each cell has a *positively charged* Nucleus, while the cell wall is *negatively charged*. This is to say that each cell uses an *electrical charge to initiate or ignite the vital cell functions* of taking in food, exporting waste and reproducing. *When fats and oils are "processed," their field of electrons have been removed and their health-giving qualities are destroyed.* The first consequence is these processed oils attach to your cell walls, blocking the insulin receptors needed to allow food/glucose into the cell. The glucose is forced to build up in the bloodstream. The second consequence is that your *cell's "battery" loses its electrical charge and is unable to ignite normal cell functions.* As you now know, high blood sugar is just a symptom of a much bigger problem.

- **One way or the other, every cell of your body is being profoundly affected by the type of fat that you eat.**

"The Battery of Life"…

Our bodies have the relentless task of making about 500 million new cells a day. This function occurs through cell division. For cell division to be successful, the new cell must

312

contain the proper amount *of electron-rich fatty acids (Good Fat)* in its cell wall to divide off from the parent cell. To be clear, every one of our trillions of cells uses an *"bioelectrical charge" to ignite vital cell functions. Without good, electron-rich fat, the crucial cell reproduction process is interrupted, or stopped. No new cells can be made, and the body begins to break down.*

In 1952, Dr. Budwig was Germany's Senior Government Expert on Fats and Pharmaceutical Drugs. Her extensive research has shown that processed fats and oils have an enormously harmful effect on our cells in two main ways: They not only severely damage our cell membrane (outer wall) but they also greatly *disrupt the electrical charge* of the cell. Let's put it this way: Processed oils *"short out"* the cell's battery, extinguishing the *"bioelectrical spark"* that triggers vital cell functions. These damaging consequences accumulate over time. As more and more of our cells slowly sicken and die, chronic illness or disease ensue.

- **Processed oils kill your cells' electrical charge, rendering it <u>unable to ignite</u> normal life-sustaining functions. The cells become <u>"dead batteries</u>."**

Continuously high blood sugar clearly indicates that your cell walls are shut down, and that a much bigger problem is now breeding. *Eating damaging processed oils for years will ensure you have an abundance of sickly cells with dead batteries. It's pretty simple: Processed oils and trans-fats intercept the cells' ability to perform their core, life-sustaining functions.*

We all know someone who has suffered the unfortunate effect of diabetes. This usually begins peripheral nerve damage (neuropathy) in their extremities, and sadly, can lead to amputation of their toes, feet or leg. *How does this happen?* The cells in those extremities have been starved to death, causing the eventual death of the limb.

Oxygen Deficiency of the Cell...
Oxygen has the ability to combine with almost any other element in the body to form vital components for sustaining life.

We have discussed at length the body's need for oxygen in every aspect of its function, small and large. oxygen is absorbed by our red blood cells (hemoglobin) and transported to every area of the body. It provides life and energy to every living cell.

We learned that in 1931, Dr. Otto Warburg won the Nobel Prize in Biochemistry for his discovery that *cancer cannot grow in a high oxygen* environment. He attests the *primary cause of cancer is the slowing down or the stopping of normal oxygen respiration by the cell. He further proved that a cell that is deprived of just 35% of its required oxygen becomes a breeding ground for disease and cancer.*

Dr. Budwig agrees.

How Tumors Develop...
According to Dr. Budwig, tumors develop when the normal growth process of the cell has been stopped or disrupted. Tumors normally occur in high growth areas of the body, such as skin, glands, liver, pancreas, stomach and intestines. Her research showed that *when the electrical charge of the cell is missing due to the lack of Electron-Rich Fat, the process of cell growth is interrupted. Because electrically active fats are not present in the cell wall, the cell substance becomes inactive, like a "dead battery,"*

314

preventing the shedding and replacing of old cells. This results in the formation of most tumors. (Budwig, 1957)

The Budwig Protocol...

Dr. Budwig discovered a groundbreaking way to reverse the stagnation of the growth process, shrink tumors and resuscitate dying cells, with a potent combination of 2 simple foods. Her exhaustive research proved there exists a unique oil (Good Fat) which was "electrically charged" and had the ability to bind with a Sulfur and Protein rich food to "reignite" the cell's battery. This simple but potent mixture was shown to easily carry needed nutrients into the smallest of capillaries and even into sick and dying cancerous cells. It was a life-changing breakthrough.

- *Her miracle recipe consists of combining Flaxseed Oil (an essential electron-rich fat) with Cottage Cheese, which is rich in Sulfur and Protein.*

The combination of these 2 foods causes a chemical reaction that makes this nutrient rich mixture generate an electromagnetic charge which is readily absorbed into a sick cell's membrane. Her exhaustive studies proved that this simple mixture recharges the "dead battery cells," in effect, resuscitating them, so they can resume normal healthy functions. Her studies confirm that once these cells are resuscitated, tumors begin to dissolve and disease symptoms reverse.

Her life-saving protocol was used to successfully treat cancer patients around the world. She attests that even patients diagnosed with terminal cancer who were sent home to die had been resuscitated by way of her Protocol. Her records confirm that she has also successfully used her treatment on Patients with MS and other chronic diseases.

Dr. Budwig asserts that, "No cell function or brain function can take place without Electron-Rich Fat. Without any doubt, it has been scientifically proven that every function of the brain needs the activation effects of Electron-Rich Fats. The same applies to nerve cells and the regeneration of muscle tissue during the oxidative recovery phase during sleep. This process requires highly saturated and unsaturated fats, particularly the Electron-Rich Fatty acids in Flaxseed Oil. So when I wish to help a very sick Patient, I must first give the most optimal Oil I have. My opinion is Flaxseed Oil." (Budwig, 1957)

Budwig Protocol Wins in Court:
"Findings Conclusive"…

Back in the day, Dr. Budwig made a lot of waves by asserting that cancerous tumors should NOT be treated with the medical standard of chemotherapy or radiation. She was brave enough to confirm this on the radio so that the sick and dying can become aware of a safer, more effective treatment for Cancer. When Dr. Budwig declared her life-changing discoveries, Germany's esteemed "Central Committee for Cancer Research" unanimously rejected her findings. They actually took her to court to rebuff her discovery as untrue. After a thorough investigation, the Judge's verdict was as follows: "Dr. Budwig's documents and papers are conclusive. There will be a scandal in the scientific world, because the public would certainly support Dr. Budwig." (Budwig, 1957)

Let's pause here to note that there are current Medical opinions that generally pooh-pooh Dr. Budwig's simple Protocol as being ineffective. Some Doctors and websites reject the Budwig Protocol by alleging "there is no

316

documentation that it works." Well, let's ask your common sense to weigh in here: *In order to be nominated for a Nobel Prize, don't you think Dr. Budwig had to produce verified documentation for all her discoveries? Don't you think she had to show scientific evidence that her simple protocol was in fact successful in healing cancer patients...? So then I'm guessing she would have surely been required to show a boatload of verification before she was nominated SEVEN TIMES for a Nobel Prize. So, I have one question for all the mockers out there: Where's THEIR Nobel Prize...?*
...just sayin'.

The Short Version:
Four Main Causes of Disease and Cancer...
  ➢ *The cell can't eat: No food can get in.*
  ➢ *The cell can't breathe: No oxygen can get in.*
  ➢ *The cell can't eject toxins: Toxins build up inside.*
  ➢ *The cell's Battery is dead: No electrical charge exists to ignite cell function.*
  ➢ *Cell can't grow normally or reproduce*

The Budwig Protocol enabling cells to:
  ➢ *Receive nutrients, eat again.*
  ➢ *Receive oxygen, breathe again.*
  ➢ *Heal cell wall, eject toxins again.*
  ➢ *Restart cell's battery to resume normal functions again.*
  ➢ *Resumes normal growth and reproduction*

The Budwig Protocol is a simple, safe alternative cancer treatment that can be life-changing for you or your loved one. *Holistic Cancer Treatments* can be the first treatment choice, before any Chemo or Radiation has damaged the body.

- *Dr. Budwig has discovered and proven that this particular combination of Good Electron-Rich Fat in Flaxseed Oil with the Calcium, Sulfur and Protein in the Cottage Cheese <u>creates a powerful electromagnetic charge</u>.*

- *This Budwig Protocol mixture easily penetrates the wall of a sick or dying cancerous cell, resuscitates it with crucial nutrients and reignites the bioelectrical charge required to resume normal healthy cell life. Summarily, reversing symptoms.*

Circa 1950-1960, there was also a *Budwig Diet* created. Dr. Budwig attested that she believed the following foods would *promote sickness and disease:*
- ➢ Margarine and all processed and hydrogenated Oils
- ➢ Ham and Bacon
- ➢ Cold Cuts and Processed Meats
- ➢ Sugar
- ➢ Processed Grains and Cereals
- ➢ Many processed Dairy Products

This list of foods was her way of *"plugging the holes in your boat"* so that your body can thoroughly heal. In other words, you can't expect the Budwig Protocol or any other method to properly heal your body if you continue to eat damaging processed oils, processed meats and excessive amounts of sugar.

Historically, the Budwig Protocol has had a very high success rate worldwide, even resuscitating cancer Patients who were diagnosed as having only days left to live. Sadly, many other Patients were already too badly damaged from radiation and chemotherapy to be saved. *The records show that for many Patients, Dr. Budwig had to administer 500 cc's of her mixture via enema, as they were too sick to even swallow. Initially, many of her Patients could not urinate or have bowel movements or even cough. But her records reflect that after receiving her Protocol, a "reactivation of their vital functions happened in many cases, with the Patient feeling immediately better."*

Dr. Budwig is quoted as saying, *"I flatly declare that the usual hospital treatments today, in the case of a tumorous growth, most certainly leads to a worsening of the disease or a speedier death."*

(Budwig, J., International Congress of Nutrition Symposium. Paris,1957.)

Let's Sum it Up…

70 years ago, Dr. Budwig discovered and proved that Processed Vegetable Oils and processed fats are one of the main causes of Cancer because they do 2 damaging things: they shut down the cell wall, disabling its ability to receive food and oxygen and to eject toxins. They also extinguish the electrical charge of the cell causing it to become a "dead battery" preventing it from reproducing normally.

The Budwig Protocol's simple Flaxseed recipe has been proven to:
- *Enter a diseased or cancerous cell to feed it.*
- *Restore cell wall permeability so diseased cell can respirate again.*
- *Create a bioelectrical charge to re-ignite the cell's battery. Cell then resumes normal cell growth and reproduction.*

- *Resuscitate dying and diseased cells, shrink tumors*

For these life-changing and documented discoveries, Dr. Budwig was nominated <u>7 times for a Nobel Prize</u>.
So yes, let's go with that.

Testimonials…

Using the Budwig Protocol, Cancer Researcher Mike Vrentas successfully cured his own wife of cancer. She is still cancer free today.

Mike is a member of the Independent Cancer Research Foundation. Following his wife's successful healing, Mike went on to develop the Cellect-Budwig Protocol. He then partnered with cancertutor.com and created the "Cellect-Budwig & More" video series, which teaches Alternative Cancer Protocols.

He developed these practices after treating many cases of cancer in all stages, learning firsthand what was most effective and what was not. For 17 years, he taught and coached more than 1,000 cancer patients all over the world. His extensive research results and personal testimony are compiled into a 25-module course teaching the Cellect-Budwig Protocol. Mike Vrentas attests this Alternative Cancer Protocol is fast-acting, effective and does not damage or harm any healthy tissue. He concludes by affirming that this treatment has demonstrated a very high percentage of positive results, not in months or weeks, but in days.

I eat the Budwig Protocol Mixture at least 3x a month. Because it is also a preventative. It keeps all my cell batteries charged and optimized.

And…I like the way it tastes.

NEXT ACTION:
 "Follow the Recipe"
   ...1,2,3...

1). The Budwig Protocol Recipe:
   ⅓ Cup of (organic) Flaxseed Oil (with Lignans is best)
   ⅔ Cup of Cottage Cheese
   1   Handful of fresh ripe Pineapple, cubed

   ➢ In a Food Processor on a LOW setting, mix the Flaxseed Oil with Cottage Cheese till well blended.

   ➢ Add a handful of fresh ripe Pineapple, cubed.

   ➢ Blend on LOW until it becomes the consistency of pudding.

   ➢ Eat within 30 minutes.

2). Eat several times a week if you are seriously sick.

3). Or eat 3-4x a month as a preventative.

The Budwig Protocol may appear to be just pineapple pudding;

   but actually
      ...it's Science.

Chapter Nine

CLEAN OUT YOUR ARTERIES
Cardio Protegen
Cardiovascular Repair & Support

I have to pause here to chuckle at myself. As my Family would tell you, for decades now, I have been singing the praises of *Cardio Protegen* to anyone with ears. And for darn good reason. I have never seen it fail to improve the health of anyone who listened. The word *Protegen* is derived from the verb *Proteger* which means "*to protect or support.*" Having over 100 active ingredients that protect and support the heart and cardio-vascular system, you now know how *Cardo Protegen* got its name.

What is it ...?
Cardio Protegen is a potent liquid supplement that looks like and tastes like cherry cough syrup. However, in actuality, is a potent combination of 19 Vitamins, 2,000 mg of ionic minerals, 1,000 mg of Omega 3's, Resveratrol, OPC Grape Seed extract and CoQ 10, Amino Acids including L-Citrulline and a whopping 5,000 mg of L-Arginine.

What do all ingredients things do...?
Omega-3...

is an Essential Fatty Acid with multiple benefits. It has been proven to improve eye health, as one of the major structural components of the eye contains a form of Omega-3. The promotion of brain health is another powerful benefit it delivers. The brain is composed of 40% DHA fatty acids; the retina of the eye is 60% DHA fatty acids. *This DHA is a type of Omega-3.*

The National Institute of Health confirms that infants fed formula fortified with DHA have better eyesight than those fed formulas without it. They further attest that enough Omega-3 during pregnancy has been linked to many benefits to the child, such as, higher intelligence, better communication and social skills, decreased risk of ADHD and Autism.

The World Health Organization confirms that Omega-3 improves numerous heart disease risk factors. Finally, it has been shown to reduce insulin resistance and protect the body against inflammation.

Grape Seed Extract…

is a powerful antioxidant. Research shows it is a major anti-inflammatory and free radical scavenger. *Providing 50x the antioxidant capacity of Vitamin E.*

CoEnzyme Q-10 (CoQ10)...

is required by every cell in the human body. It is needed to help produce energy needs of the body through the production of ATP (energy molecule). Extensive studies have shown that CoQ10 can revitalize the heart, the Immune System and cellular function.

Resveratrol…

is the bioflavonoid antioxidant found in the skin of red grapes. One ounce of Cardio Protegen has the Resveratrol equivalent of 115 glasses of red wine.

L-Arginine / Heavyweight Healer…

is a naturally occurring Amino Acid that is a "vaso-dialator" which means it naturally dilates the blood vessels. This is a crucial action for people with high blood pressure and arteriosclerosis. These people are most likely taking prescription drugs to dilate their blood vessels but are also incurring harmful side effects from those drugs. *Science has proven that L-Arginine naturally reduces arterial plaque, unclogs arteries, lowers high blood pressure, prevents blood clots, lowers cholesterol, and improves heart performance.*

L-Citrulline and L-Arginine…

are synergistically powerful for Nitric Oxide production, which has been shown to prevent and reverse arterial plaque buildup and improves heart function and cardiovascular health.

The benefits of all these Vitamins and minerals are well known; but it is the *synergistic combination* of them with the L-Arginine and L-Citrulline that makes this supplement both unique and powerful.

Anginarex.com confirms "Cardio Protegen has been thoroughly tested and was found to deliver very impressive results to its users."

The Harmful Effects of Cholesterol-Lowering Statin Drugs…

Statin Drugs have been shown to cause liver, kidney and muscle damage. They block the body's production of CoQ10 which is needed for energy and proper function of every cell. Cholesterol lowering drugs in fact deplete the body of necessary *Good Fats* which are vital for hormone production, cell wall integrity and especially for the proper function of the brain cells. In the *Alzheimer's Chapter (Chapter 7)* we discussed at length the consequences suffered by brain cells when it is deprived of *Good Fat.*

The body needs Good Cholesterol and Good Fat to maintain optimal health and function. Good Cholesterol actually used to protect cells and support heart and arteries. The body actually manufactures its own Cholesterol as needed for vital functions. *Statin Drugs do NOT differentiate between Good Fat and Bad Fat,* or between Good Cholesterol and Bad Cholesterol. *They deplete all of them.* This depletion of Good Fat causes an entire universe of new problems for the Patient.

As you previously learned, arterial plaque is made up of Calcium, fibrin, cholesterol and waste products. This mixture is produced by the body in response to injuries to the arterial walls. As advised, like a *Biological Band-Aid,* this mixture is used to "*patch injuries*" on the arterial wall. Over time, the accumulation of these patches cause the narrowing of that artery. Specifically, it is the Calcium that contributes to the *hardening* of the artery. Injuries to the arterial walls are the result of free radical damage and microbial attack or infection. *You can see why just trying to chemically reduce all the fat in the body is NOT the healthy or permanent solution to atherosclerosis or high blood pressure.*

Dr. Harry's Case History
Cardiovascular System Rejuvenated…

The very first video I watched about Cardio Protegen (then *Mega Cardio*) sold me. One of Cardio Protegen's Inventors, Dr. Harry, attested that *we are as old as our cardiovascular system.* He explained how Japanese hospitals use a medical device that measures the age of the

Patient's cardiovascular system. He obtained this device for the purpose of showing changes in the cardiovascular system after taking Cardio Protegen.

What he first discovered alarmed him. His own cardiovascular system tested much older than his biological age, as did his daughter and his friend, who was a football player and an athlete. All three of them started taking Cardio Protegen. *A few months later when retested, it was proven that all three of their cardiovascular systems had literally reversed in measurable age markers and were greatly increased in health markers, including much improved cholesterol levels and blood pressure.*

...I was in.

Coronary Bypass Surgery Canceled...

It was this next testimonial that shocked me. Dr. Harry was on a talk show relaying how he had gone to a wedding and met an elderly man named Don who was scheduled for triple bypass surgery. The Doctor had advised that Don's *arteries were 90% blocked.* Upon learning this, Dr. Harry urged Don to take Cardio Protegen liquid supplement 3x a day (that is 3 ounces), as this man's condition was severe.

Each month, Don's test results improved. Within 3 months, the Cardiologist *canceled the bypass surgery, declaring that Dan's tests showed his arteries were now 90% CLEAR.*

...Oh yes. I was DEFINITELY in.

TESTIMONIALS:

I have two very powerful and very personal victory stories about this product, which is why I am its *biggest fan.*

PERMANENTLY REVERSED FATHER'S DIABETES
83-Year-Old, Eliminates 5 Prescriptions

In 2007, I first learned about *Cardio Protegen* which was then called *Mega Cardio.* At that time, my 83-year-old Father was diabetic and was taking 5 prescription drugs: insulin stimulating pills (3x a day), blood thinners, beta blockers, cholesterol reducing drugs, and blood pressure medication. He had his blood work done every 3 months *to monitor whether his liver and kidney functions were failing due to all these drugs.* It made no sense to me that he was prescribed drugs that would eventually terminally damage his liver and kidneys.

I started him on Cardio Protegen, 1 liquid ounce per day on an empty stomach and no food for 1-2 hours afterwards. We checked his blood sugar and blood pressure each week. As his improvements progressed, we incrementally weaned him off of his medications accordingly.

At the end of three months, he was off all medications. At the end of four months he went to Dr. Jones for his blood test. She was flabbergasted. She said "*all his* numbers were *better than normal!*" Pop confessed to her that he stopped taking all her prescriptions 4 months ago. She replied, *"Well, whatever you are doing, keep doing it!"* She wanted to retest him in 30 days to confirm his "healing" was permanent.

Thirty days later, Dr. Jones did a second blood test on Pop. She declared that all Pop's numbers remained stable and healthy. At that point, she called me at home to ask, "WHAT are you giving you Father? In all my years as a Doctor, I have never before declared anyone 'no longer a diabetic', let alone an 83-year-old man! Please tell me what you are giving him, as my Mother is severely diabetic…and I can't help her."

I admired Dr. Jones for having the intelligence and receptivity to accept that a safe and successful healing had happened to her Patient, with results so remarkable that she wanted that same therapy for her own Mother.

The need for Pop's blood-thinning drugs was eliminated, because the Cardio Protegen, naturally corrects blood viscosity (thickness). This lessens the likelihood of blood clots and the likelihood of stroke caused by blood clots. You see now how correcting one disorder leads to the natural correction of others. Because Cardio Protegen strengthens and assists in the repair of the entire cardiovascular system, heart function is greatly improved eliminating the need for Beta Blockers. The ingredients in Cardio Protegen clean plaque from the arteries, eliminating the need for high cholesterol and high blood pressure drugs. His pancreas stimulating pills were eliminated, because *Pop's blood sugar was stabilized without medication…for the rest of his life.*
This was the first life-changing event that made me believe in Cardio Protegen.

TAKEN OFF HEART DONOR'S LIST
75-Year-Old Man, Heart Function Restored
Peter was a friend of mine. He was 75 years old and very overweight. He had the stereotypical ill health consisting of high cholesterol, high blood pressure, thickened blood and diabetes. He was taking a plethora of prescriptions. One day he told me that his Doctor advised him that his heart was *only functioning at 25%.* The Doctor recommended that Peter be put on the Heart Donors list; but cautioned Peter's wife to be prepared, as it was very probable that Peter would just die in his sleep before he ever receives a new heart. Peter and his wife were devastated by this news. I asked him to please

start taking Cardio Protegen immediately, as it was specifically formulated *to repair and rejuvenate the cardiovascular system.* I instructed that he take 1 ounce 3x a day (instead of once a day) as his condition was dire. This was June, 2009.

By the end of September 2009, 4 months later, Peter was removed from the Heart Donors List. His Cardiologist advised his heart was now functioning at 75%!

This second life-changing event sealed it for me, and I hope for you. I have witnessed that, taken correctly, Cardio Protegen has the powerful ability to clean out arteries, balance blood viscosity, lower blood pressure, rejuvenating and strengthening the heart and the Cardiovascular System.

...and now you know why

I am its biggest Fan.

NEXT ACTION:
 "Follow the Recipe" ...1,2,3...

- Take 1 liquid ounce of Cardio Protegen in 8 ounces of water, at least 3 hours after any food (best to take first thing in the morning or last thing before bed).

- MUST TAKE ON AN EMPTY STOMACH

- MUST NOT EAT FOR 2 HOURS AFTERWARDS.
  The strongest ingredients in this product are Amino Acids. These wrestle with the Amino Acids that are in food. So if you take this product with any food or drink or within 2 hours of a meal, you will LESSEN ITS EFFECT and waste your money and your time. *So please, Follow the Recipe.*

329

RESOURCES:

To Order Cardio Protegen:
  352-567-0002 (9:00am to 5:00pm EST)
Each 32 oz bottle should last one month.
Can also get 1 oz travel size bottles.
Cost: Approximately $48.00 per month.
Autoship cost is less, plus free shipping.

(…No, I do not sell this product. I only love it.)

Chapter Ten

RECHARGE THE BATTERY OF LIFE
CELLFOOD

CELLFOOD
Deeply Detoxes and Electrically Supercharges Every Cell while Infusing Hydrogen and Oxygen into the Body.

CellFood is a liquid supplement that has the slight taste of lemon. Inside this seemingly simple liquid exists a universe of health-giving properties.

It is a proprietary ionic, colloidal suspension consisting of dissolved oxygen, 78 ionic minerals, 34 enzymes and 17 amino acids. It has been formulated to achieve maximum cell oxygenation. When mixed with water, Cellfood produces both oxygen and hydrogen. When ingested, it then delivers all the above life-giving nutrients into the blood and into every cell in the body, substantially increasing Cellular Respiration.

The overall results of this are increased cellular metabolism, strength and energy. This substantially increases each cell's ability to continually eject toxins, powerfully detoxing the body as a whole

Bottom line, it turns your every Cell into a veritable Powerhouse.

Cellular Respiration…
The BEST Detox in Town…

- ***Cellfood activates Optimal Cellular Respiration which deeply detoxifies every cell.***

Believe me. *You can drink green smoothies til you TURN green. But if the electromagnetic charge of your cell is "off," then you are beating a dead horse. We learned in Chapter 8 that if your cell battery is dead, then proper cell function and respiration is disabled. This results in sickness and disease.*

Simply put, Cellular Respiration is the ability of the cell to *"breathe in"* oxygen and nutrients and to *"breathe out"* waste and toxins. This is its basic life function. <u>*It is both fundamental and crucial that all of our cells are respiring at full capacity*</u>. As discussed, if the individual cells weaken or malfunction due to lack of proper "food in, waste out" function, a downward spiral domino effect begins, triggering sickness and disease throughout the entire body.

<u>*When Cellular Respiration is at its peak, the cell deeply and automatically detoxes itself, with every "cellular exhale" (ejection of toxins and waste)*</u>. *So, by supercharging Cell Respiration, you turn your every cell into a high-performance, "self-cleaning furnace," purring along in power and health.*

Now, just multiply that times 37 trillion cells.

What Does Cellfood Do…?

- *Cellfood produces both oxygen and hydrogen in the body. Hydrogen and oxygen sustain all life on Earth.*

- *Cellfood gives a high electrostatic charge to every cell. This ignites & maintains its electrical charge.*

- *It ignites deep cellular detox through acute ejection of toxins.*

Cellfood gives Oxygen:
Oxygen Deficiency is the Primary Cause of Cell Death / Disease...

Oxygen has been called *"the Giver of Life."* Our body is composed of 65% Oxygen (O_2.) Oxygen is the fuel that powers every cell in our body, enabling them to perform at optimal capacity. Every cell in our body requires O_2 to metabolize food, eliminate waste, to heal, regenerate and to reproduce. Oxygen has the unique ability of combining with almost every other element to form biological actions that are crucial for the life of the cell and the body. Proteins are formed when O_2 binds with nitrogen, carbon and hydrogen. Proteins are needed to build and maintain healthy body tissues. When O_2 binds with hydrogen and carbon, carbohydrates are formed which the body uses for physical energy.

We are urged to "hydrate" after a workout. This is because the water (H_2O) you drink breaks down into *hydrogen and oxygen* in the body. Oxygen is then absorbed by the hemoglobin (red blood cells) and delivered to every cell. Low oxygen causes poor stamina, fatigue, cell inefficiency and sickness. A lack of oxygen promotes cancer, disease and cell death.

In previous chapters, we have discussed at length that oxygen is the primary healing and energy-giving element in the body. *Molecular Biologist Stephen Levine asserts that oxygen deficiency is the single greatest cause of all disease. oxygen deficiency accompanies and is an integral aspect of all disease states.*

By now, you may feel like Dr. Otto Warburg is a close friend, as we have visited his life-changing discoveries several times, as follows:

In 1931, renowned Biochemist Dr. Otto Warburg was awarded the Nobel Prize for his discovery that cancer and disease breed in a low oxygen environment. His discovery confirmed that when cell oxygen level falls, that cell begins to fester and ferment, opening the door for cancer.

- *He attested that if a healthy cell is deprived of just 35% of its required oxygen, it becomes a breeding ground for cancer.*

- *This powerful discovery confirmed that the opposite is also true. That is to say, a body that is high in oxygen is resistant to cancer and most diseases. This is why Oxygen Therapy has been used for 150 years to treat sickness and disease. Because for all the above reasons, oxygen heals and prevents disease.*

Biochemist David Holden has practiced *Preventative Natural Medicine* for 30 years. He confirms that "*Stabilized oxygen is a welcome arrival to any therapist looking for effective solutions to accelerate treatment programs.*" *Oxygen is a powerful detoxifier.* When it is deficient, microbes and toxins take root and begin to overtake the cells, eventually prevailing over the body.

Oxygen Therapy is any method that increases oxygen in the body or that increases the absorption of oxygen by the body. Some are complicated like the Hyperbaric Chamber and intravenous Ozone (O3) Therapy. But fortunately, there are other methods of oxygenating the body that are simple, safe and very effective. They are: *Essential Oils (Chapter 2), Food Grade Hydrogen Peroxide (Chapter 5), and Cellfood Drops.*

We focus here on Cellfood Drops. When added to water, it is important to note that Cellfood generates and delivers nascent (newborn) oxygen, O2 atoms and hydrogen, H2 atoms to the blood and to every cell in the body. It does not create free radicals, but in fact binds to them and creates even more stable oxygen. *In this simple but profound mechanism, Cellfood powerfully charges, oxygenates and invigorates every cell in the body, while also increasing the rate at which the cells eject waste and toxins.*

- **By simply taking 7 drops of Cellfood in a glass of water twice daily, your cells can detox on automatic pilot.**

Cellfood also gives Hydrogen:
 What does Hydrogen Bring to the Party...?
 Hydrogen makes up about 90% of all atoms and 75% of the mass of the Universe. *It is considered "the Master Builder."* The stars are made of hydrogen. The sun is a giant ball of hydrogen and helium gasses. These gasses combine to form helium atoms in a process called *Fusion* which gives off massive amounts of *Radiant Energy.* Hydrogen contains the highest energy of any fuel by weight. Its energy is stored in fossil fuels. This *Radiant Energy*

335

causes plants to grow. *It is found in all living things. It sustains all life on Earth.*

Hydrogen is required to perform most bodily processes. It is a crucial part of the *electron transport chain* which is a series of chemical reactions that create energy/ATP inside the cell. Hydrogen is critical for the building and repair of cells, organs and the body's Immune System. In the body, the actions of hydrogen are balanced by oxygen.

The inventor of Cellfood, Everett Storey affirms, *"The winding road to health leads ever uphill from some form of hydrogen, which is about to be recognized as the creative and sustaining force of all life."*

- *Cellfood is the simplest known method of Hydrogen and Oxygen Therapy.*

Long History of Cellfood:
Water purifier…

Developed in the 1940s, Cellfood was found to be a very potent bacteriostatic (having the ability to inhibit bacterial growth). In 1956, it was used as a drinking water purifier for the Military. Putting 20 drops of Cellfood into a gallon of water and letting it sit for 6 hours resulted in clean drinking water.

Metabolic Efficiency Catalyst…

Cellfood's unique formula contains trace minerals as well as activated digestive and metabolic enzymes. This increases cell metabolism and enhances the absorption of all nutrients. It further promotes greater absorption and bioavailability of vitamins, minerals and nutrient factors.

Balances Metabolism in Cells and Tissue…

Cellfood's formula is highly *electrostatically charged*, that is, it has an abundance of electrons. It also has a *bipolar valence or capacity*. This brings a unique two-fold treatment to cell and tissue imbalance. In short, Cellfod is able to act as an *Adaptogen* in this regard, by *correcting both anabolic or catabolic imbalance.*

Free Radicals Scavenger…

Cellfood has a unique "water splitting technology." When added to water, Cellfood splits the water molecule creating nascent *(newborn) Oxygen Atoms.* In Biochemical terms, this newborn Oxygen Atom is negatively charged (O). It is believed that one of the primary causes of degenerative disease and aging is Free Radicals, which are positively charged single atoms of oxygen (O+). The new Oxygen Atom from Cellfood combines with the Free Radical Atom *to form a pure Oxygen* (O_2) molecule at the cellular level where it is most needed. This pure O_2 molecule can then bind with carbon waste forming carbon dioxide (CO_2), which is easily exhaled from the body.

Many Patients have reported that they have less sickness and nausea from chemo and radiation when they are using Cellfood.

Increased Energy…

Successfully delivering extra oxygen, hydrogen, enzymes and Amino Acids into each cell substantially increases cellular efficiency resulting in overall increased energy to the body. Designed as an ionic formula within a colloidal suspension, Cellfood has the powerful capacity to easily replenish the blood levels of these nutrients.

337

Natural Microbe Repellent...

Specifically, the infusion of each cell with oxygen and hydrogen creates a high oxygen state within each cell, which strongly repels the attack and growth of bacteria, viruses, fungi and parasites.

Tissue Healer...

Cellfood acts as a Donor of free electrons. It has the ability to disinfect wounds and to initiate issue repair on contact at a cellular level.

Balances the Body's pH...

Regardless if the body is too alkaline or too acidic, test results confirm that Cellfood brings the body into a balanced neutral pH of approximately 7.0.

Delivers High Frequency &
 Electromagnetic Charge to the Cells...

When Cellfood's *"water splitting phenomenon"* takes place, *an enormous supply of positively-charged electromagnetic energy is created. It is through this mechanism that Cellfood raises the Frequency of all organs in the body.* This specifically strengthens the Immune System. You learned in Chapter 2 how *Frequency* is the measure of Electrical Energy in the body. *The higher the body's Frequency, the more difficult it is for pathogens to live or breed there. We learned, a low Frequency body invites systemic infections and disease.*

Boosts Immune System...

In 1991, Dr. Aristo Vojdani, Vice President of Immusciences Laboratories Inc. USA reported that the *body's production of germ-fighting T-Cells were significantly*

338

increased when the dosage of Cellfood was increased. This confirmed that the Immune System was being progressively strengthened by the ingestion of Cellfood.

Supercharge the Battery of Life…

One drop of Cellfood produces 77,000 Angstroms of Energy. This, in conjunction with an infusion of oxygen and hydrogen, turbocharges and powerfully detoxes every cell

Cellfood is a proprietary formula of pure ionic trace minerals, enzymes and amino acids. It uniquely mimics the body's extracellular fluid, having similar mineral composition. Cellfood nutrients are readily and efficiently absorbed at the cellular level, as they are amazingly small, 4-7 nanometers in size. This enables Cellfood to pass very easily through the cell wall, bringing nutrients, oxygen and hydrogen *IN, and* throwing toxins and waste *OUT. The optimization of this process strengthens and balances the Whole Body System…*

- Brings physical strength via essential minerals and amino acids needed for a healthy body constitution.

- Brings *Electrical Balance* via raising Frequency in organs and nervous system and keeping the "battery charged" in every cell.

- Boosts Immunity via oxygen, hydrogen and Frequency.

- Enhances Digestive and Metabolic processes via Enzymes.

- Establishes and maintains *Optimal Cell Respiration and Detoxification.*

- Promotes the health, vitality and longevity of every cell.

The Short Version…

Cellfood has been successfully used for over 60 years in 90 countries around the world. It champions the unique ability of powerfully detoxing the body at the deepest cellular level. It delivers a high hydrogen and oxygen to the body. It raises the body's Frequency. It also bioelectrically recharges every cell, causing optimal Respiration and deep Cellular Detox.

In short, Cellfood causes each cell to become a supercharged, high performing, "self-cleaning" machine.

THE SUM OF ALL WELLNESS WISDOM…
Here's what you've learned
on your WELLNESS WARRIOR journey:

"Plug the Holes in Your Boat"...
Allow Optimal Healing by REMOVING:
- ➢ **ALL PROCESSED OR HYDROGENATED OILS AND FATS!**
- ➢ *The Dirty Dozen/Top 12 Avoid Foods for your specific Blood Type.*
- ➢ *Amalgam (silver) fillings; replace with Composite filling.*
- ➢ *Root canal teeth; can be replaced with implants.*
- ➢ *Nickel bridges; and replace with porcelain.*

"Follow the Recipe"...
Achieve Optimal Health & Vitality by ADDING:
- ➢ *4-8 Tablespoons of <u>unrefined</u> Coconut Oil every day. Cook with it. Use it as butter on everything. Put into smoothies. In your hot drinks.*
- ➢ *1-2 drops of Essential Oils applied to throat glands & chest each morning and before bed.*
- ➢ *20 minutes of Oil Pulling each day.*
- ➢ *5-7 drops of Cellfood in cup of water 1-2x each day.*
- ➢ *A Food Grade H2O2 bath twice a week; or use in a vaporizer or in a 3% solution nasal spray or on your toothbrush.*

What Natural and Holistic Therapies can Penetrate, Feed and most often Resuscitate a Sick or Diseased Cell…
- ➢ *Coconut Oil via Medium Chain Fatty Acids*
- ➢ *Essential Oils via Oxygen & High Frequency*
- ➢ *Hydrogen Peroxide via Oxygen*

- *Budwig Protocol via Medium Chain Fatty Acids, Protein, Sulfur + Electromagnetic Charge*
- *Cardio Protegen via Ionic Minerals, L-Arginine, Plant compounds*
- *Cellfood via Oxygen, Hydrogen, Enzymes & Electromagnetic Charge*

Natural Paths to Deep Cellular Detox:
Simple and Powerful...

1) Coconut Oil
2) Oil Pulling
3) Essential Oils
4) Food Grade Hydrogen Peroxide
5) Cellfood Drops

What Three Things can Kill a Virus...

By now, you have learned that there are only 3 things in this world that can safely kill a Virus and most other pathogens: Unrefined Coconut Oil, Pure Therapeutic Grade Essential Oils and Food Grade Hydrogen Peroxide (oxygen). From your journey through this book, you are now well informed on all of them.

...Yay for you!

Each of these life-giving practices dramatically rivet every cell to its highest performance capacity, shifting it into its optimal level of strength and vitality.

If you use any combination of these potent protocols every day, you will be keeping your cells Supercharged and deeply Detoxed, not once...but for a lifetime.

This applies to brain cells, heart cells, blood cells
...ALL cells.

Are You Proactive…or Reactive…?

With regards to our health, we are a population that has become *reactive instead of being proactive.*

We wait until we are sick and then frantically scramble to regain our health. The Holistic Healing methods in this book are the safest and most powerful that I have ever experienced for healing and for prevention of sickness and disease. You have learned some *Ancient Healing Practices* that have been repeatedly proven over hundreds or thousands of years. *You have seen a deluge of documented scientific studies performed over decades of time, which verify that the proper practice of one or all of the advised Natural Healing Methods should substantially improve your overall health and vitality in safe and simple ways.*

<u>*Down the Rabbit Hole*</u>*…*

Do you feel like you're headed down the Rabbit Hole of taking more and more prescription drugs that don't seem to be helping but in fact are making you feel weaker?

You have now accumulated enough knowledge to make an informed choice of a much better path to health. It's a life-changing choice.

At this journey's end, you have assembled an arsenal of powerful Healing and Wellness Wisdom from which to choose, as follows: Unrefined Coconut Oil, Therapeutic Essential Oils, Oil Pulling, Food Grade Hydrogen Peroxide, Cardio Protegen, Cellfood drops, "Blood Type Diet," and the Budwig Protocol.

Choose to do some of these practices,
or choose to do them all.
Realize that each one is a Brick of Wellness
in your hands.

There are several continuous themes woven through the pages of this book. One is that all of these advised *Holistic Healing Protocols* have been proven to be tremendously effective when you *FOLLOW THE RECIPE.* Next, if properly done, they have no known negative side effects. Finally, it is highly probable that *most Doctors will not believe a word of it.* They may even try to talk you out of it. Because *Natural Remedies and Healing Protocols are foreign to them.* They were *not taught* Holistic Healing in Medical School. As a result, most Doctors will usually refute what they do not know.

Please remember that several Doctors have called me at home to find out what Treatment I used to get certain amazing results for their Patients, such as: *How did we reverse Mother's Alzheimer's symptoms in 4 months?...How did we reverse my Father's diabetes and wean him off 5 prescriptions?...How did Mother's shingles disappear in 5 days and never return?... How did we dissolve away my friend's Pilonidal Cyst?…What did I give to Peter that caused his heart function to go from 25% to 75% in 4 months?...How did we get Claudia's husband out of his wheelchair and off disability after 3 years of an "incurable" sickness?*

...The list goes on.

So <u>*please don't be dissuaded*</u> *if at first your Doctor is not the head cheerleader for your Holistic Choices. Doctors are intelligent people. But, Doctors are "result oriented." Once they see a measurable and unexpected improvement in a Patient, they will usually tell that Patient, "Whatever you are doing…KEEP doing it!"*

I have heard this many times, like music to my ears.

DISCLAIMER / IMPORTANT:

- *Bear in mind that no one should ever just suddenly abandon all their medication. All the testimonials in this book advise a gradual weaning off medications week by week, as improvements manifested in the Patient by way of these Holistic Treatments.*

- *Whether following Holistic or Allopathic treatments, always <u>listen to your body</u> and never exceed your physical or emotional limits.*

- *I can't promise you will be cured of every illness or have the exact results I have advised here. But I am confident that the probability of you being stronger, healthier and on less medication is extremely high by way of these simple, all-natural Protocols; as compared to you having zero likelihood of better health if you do nothing different.*

Ultimately, what I hope you have learned on our journey is that all the many reported healings, relief and even just substantial improvement of symptoms have all resulted from very simple treatments.

When done properly, there are no negative side effects from any of these Protocols. Assuming these simple Practices are just "too good to be true" would be, in my opinion, a very grave miscalculation.

If you have learned that a Powerful Preventative and Natural Cure does NOT have to be complicated, then I have fulfilled the Intention of this Book.

You purchased this book in your search for a hidden pathway to better health that is safe, natural and simple. Some of you are hungry to learn *safe, effective ways to prevent illness and disease.* Others wake up each day hoping they will somehow find a simple cure or relief from their chronic suffering; hoping each day that *there is an easier, safer and far more effective way of rebuilding their health and their life.*

In this book, I am blessed to bring you all of the above.

It's been an honor to bring you what I believe to be the easiest and most effective Holistic Healing Practices that I have ever learned. I present them to you with my heartfelt prayer that you will now take all this new-found Wellness Wisdom and use it to your highest advantage. *Claim and maintain* your personal *best level of Health and Vitality.*

Do this for yourself. Do it for your loved ones.

Rebuild your Body; Rebuild your Life.
The tools are in your hands.

The Power Path to Ultimate Wellness and Vitality
has been forged for you.
All you have to do is Follow the Map...Follow the
Recipe.

You're only One Choice away from having the
Lifelong Health and Vitality
of a
Wellness Warrior.

If you haven't already done so, please pause here to lead others to better health, by leaving a Book Review now on Amazon.

Using just 1 minute of your time, you have the power to change someone's health and someone's life, for the better…

REFERENCES

CHAPTER 1: THE TREE OF LIFE, COCONUT OIL

Addis, P.B. G.J. Warner (1991). *Free Radicals and Food Additives.*

London: Taylor and Francis.

Baba, N. (1982). Enhanced Thermogenesis and Diminished Deposition of Fat from Overfeeding with Medium Chain Triglycerides (MCFA's).

American Journal of Clinical Nutrition 35.

Berlitz, H.D., W. Grosch. (1999). *Food Chemistry.* (2nd ed.).

New York: Springer-Verlag.

Campbell-Falck, D., T. Thomas, T.M. Falck, et al. (2000)

The Intravenous Use of Coconut Water. *American Journal of Emergency Medicine18.*

Chowhan, G.S., K.R. Yoshi, H.N. Batnager, et al. (1985).

Treatment of Tapeworms Infestation with Coconut Oil. *Journal of the Asso. of Physicians of India.*

Cohen, L.A., D.O. Thompson. (1987). *The* Influence of Medium Chain Triglycerides in Rat mammary tumor development. *Lipids 22.*

Crook, W. (1986). *The Yeast Connection.* New York: Vintage Books.

Divi, R.L., H. Chang, D.R. Doerge. (1997). Anti-Thyroid Isoflavones from Soybean Oil.

Biochemical Pharmacology 54.

Dwivedi,C., et al. (1997). Preventative Effects of Rose Essential Oil on Skin Papillomas in Mice. *European Journal of Cancer Prevention.*

Enig, M.G. (1993). Coronary Heart Disease. *London: Janis.*

Enig, M.G. (1999). Coconut: In Support of Good Health in the 21st Century. *APCC.*

Enig, M.G. (2000). *Know Your Fats.* Bethesda Press.

Fife, B. (2013). *The Coconut Oil Miracle. (5th ed.)* Penguin Group.

Geliebter, A., N. Torbay, E.F. Bracco, et al. (1983). Overfeeding with Medium Chain Fatty Acids result in Diminished Deposits of Fat.

American Journal of Clinical Nutrition 37.

Heimlich, J. (1990). *What Your Doctor Won't Tell You.* New York: Harper-Perennial.

Hernell, O., H. Ward, L. Blackberg, et al. (1986). Killing of Giardia Lamblia by Human Milk Lipase. *Journal of Infectious Diseases.*

H.L. (1989). Thermogenesis in Humans with Overfeeding with Medium Chain Triglycerides. *Metabolism 38.*

Hopkins, G.J., T.G. Kennedy, K.K. Carroll. (1981). Polyunsaturated Fats as a Promoter of Mammary

Carcinogenesis. *Journal of the National Cancer Institute 66.*

Ingle, D.L. (1999). Dietary Energy Value of Medium Chain Triglycerides.

Journal of Food Science 64.

Isaacs, C.E., H. Thormar. (1990). Human Milk Lipids Inactivated Enveloped Viruses.

Breastfeeding, Nutrition, Infection and Infant Growth. *Newfoundland: Arts Biomedical.*

Isaacs, C.E., H. Thormar. (1991). The Role of Milk Derived Antimicrobial Lipids as Antiviral and Antibacterial Agents.

Immunology of Milk and the Neonate.
New York: Plenum Press.

Isaacs, C.E., R.E. Litov, H. Thormar, et al. (1992). Addition of Lipases to Infant Formula Produces Antiviral, Antibacterial Activity. *Journal of Nutritional Biochemistry 3.*

Kabara, J.J. (1978). Fatty Acids as Antimicrobial Agents. The Pharmacological Effects of Lipids. *Journal of the American Oil Chemists' Society.*

Kabara, J.J. (1984). Antimicrobial Agents Derived from Fatty Acids.
Journal of the American Oil Chemists' Society.

Kabara, J.J. (1984). *Lauricidin: Nonionic Emulsifier with Antimicrobial Properties.*

Cosmetic and Drug Preservation Principles and Practice. New York: Marcel Dekker.

Kaunitz, H. (1986). Medium Chain Triglycerides in Aging and Arteriosclerosis.
Journal of Environmental Pathology, Toxicology and Oncology.

Montserrat, A.J., M. Romeron. Lago, et al. (1995) Protective Effect of Coconut Oil on Renal Necrosis. *Renal Failure 17.*

Parekh, P.I., A.E. Petro, J.M. Tiller, et al. (1998). Reversal of Diet-Induced Obesity and Diabetes. *Metabolism 47.*

Price, W.A. (1998). *Nutrition and Physical Degeneration.* (6th ed.) Los Angeles: Keats.

Prior, I.A. (1971). *The Price of Civilization. Nutrition Today,* July/August.

Prior, I.A., F. Davidson, C.E. Salmond, Z. Czochanski. (1981). *Cholesterol,* Coconuts and Diets on Polynesian Atolls. The Pukapuka and Tokelau Island Studies.
American Journal of Clinical Nutrition.

Ross, D.L., K.F. Swaiman, F. Torres, et al. (1985). Biochemical and EEG correlates of Ketogenic Diet in Children with Epilepsy. *Pediatric Neurology 1.*

Seaton, T.B., S.L. Welle, M.K. Warenko, et al. (1986). Thermic Effect of Medium Chain and Long Chain Fatty Acids in Man. *American Journal of Clinical Nutrition 44.*

Shepard, T.H. (1960). Soybean Goiter. *New England Journal of Medicine, 262.*

Thampan, P.K. (1994). *Facts and Fallacies About Coconut Oil.*

Jakarta: Asian and Pacific Coconut Community.

Vaidya, U.V., V.M. Hegde, S.A. Behave, et al. (1992). Coconut Oil Feed in Nutrition of Very Low Birthweight Babies. *Indian Pediatrics 29.*

Yost, T.J., R.H. Eckel. (1989). Metabolic Effects of Feeding Medium Chain Triglycerides to Obese Women. *American Journal of Clinical Nutrition 39.*

World Health Organization. (1977). *Dietary Fats and Oils In Human Nutrition.*

Report of Expert Consultation. Rome: U.N. Food and Agriculture Organization.

CHAPTER 2: THE BLOOD OF THE PLANT, ESSENTIAL OILS

Al-Awadi, F.M., et al. (1987). Antidiabetic Action of Essential Oils. *Acta Diabetol Lat.*

Benencia, F., et al. (1999). Antiviral Activity of Sandalwood Essential Oil Against Herpes Virus 1 and 2. *Phytomedicine.*

Concha, J.M., et al. (1998). Wm J. Stickel Bronze Award.

Antifungal Activity of Melaleuca Essential Oil Against Pathogenic Organisms. *J Am Podiatr Med Assoc.*

Dolara, P., et al. (1996). Analgesic Effects of Myrrh Essential Oil. *Nature, Jan 4.*

Elson, C.E., et al.(1989). Impact of Lemongrass Essential Oil on Serum Cholesterol. *Lipids.*

Essential Oils Desk Reference. (2000). Essential Science Publishing.

Fang, H.J., et al. (1989). *Studies on Chemical Components and Antitumoral Action of Essential Oils.* Yao Hsueh Pao.

Fyfe, L., et al. (1997). Inhibition of Listeria and salmonella by Plant Oils. *Int. J. Antimicrobial Agents.*

Gobel, H., et al. (1994). Effects of Peppermint Oil and Eucalyptus Oil on Neurophysiological Algesimetric Headache Parameters. *Cephalalgia.*

Guillemain, J., et al. (1989). Neuro Sedative Effects of Essential Oil Of Lavender. *Ann Pharm Fr.*

Hammer, K.A., et al. (1999). Treatment of Lactobacilli and Bacterial Vaginosis with Melaleuca Essential Oil. *Antimicrobial Agents Chemotherapy.*

Jayashree, T., et al. (1999). Antiaflatoxigenic Activity of Eugenol in Clove Essential Oil.

Letter of Applied Microbiology.

Juergens, U.R., et al. (1998). Therapeutic Use of Essential Oils in Inflammatory Disease. *European Journal of Medical Research.*

Kennedy, A. (2016). *Portable Essential Oils: Remedies for Natural Health and Wellness.* Althea Press.

Kim, H.M. et al. (1999). Essential Oil of Lavender Inhibits Immediate Allergic Reaction in Mice and Rats. *J Pharm Pharmacol.*

Lachowicz, K.L., et al. (1998). The Synergistic Preservative Effect of Essential Oil of Basil Against Food Microflora. *Journal of Applied Microbiology.*

Larrondo J.V., et al. (1995). Antimicrobial Activity of Essential Oils. *Microbios.* Lis-Balchin, M., et al. (1998). Antimicrobial Activity of Essential Oils.

Letter of Applied Microbiology.

Lis-Balchin, et al. (1998). Antibacterial Effects of Essential Oils. *Letter of Applied Microbiology.*

Lorenzetti, B.B., et al. (1995). Analgesic Action of Lemongrass Tea.

J Ethnopharmacol. Michie, C.A., et al. (1991). Frankincense and Myrrh as Remedies in Children. *Journal R Social Medicine.*

Mahmood, N., et al. (1996). Anti-HIV Activity of Essential Oil of Rose.

Biochem Biophys Res Commun.

Nishijima, H., et al. (1999). Vasorelaxation Action of Eugenol in Clove Essential Oil.

Japan Journal of Pharmacology.

Pattnaik, S., et al. (1996). Antibacterial and Antifungal Activities of Ten Essential Oils.

Microbios. Reddy, B.S., et al. (1997). Prevention of Colon Carcinogenesis. *Cancer Res.*

Samman, M.A., et al. (1998). Peppermint Essential Oil prevents Carcinogenesis in Hamsters. *Carcinogenesis.*

Syed, T.A., et al. (1999). Treatment of Toenail Fungus with Melaleuca Essential Oil.

Trop Med Int Health.

Sysoev, N.P. (1991). Effects of Essential Oils on Blood Neutrophils in Mucosa Trauma

of the Mouth. *Stomatologija.* Tantaoui-Elaraki, A., et al. (1994). Inhibition of Growth and Aflatoxin Production by

Essential Oils. *Journal of Environmental Pathology, Toxicology and Oncology.*

Tovey, E.R., et al. (1997). Eucalyptus Oil for Controlling Dust Mites and Allergens.

Journal Allergy Clinical Immunol.

Wan, J., et al. (1998). The Effects of Essential Oil of Basil on the Growth of Aeromonas Hydrophila. *Journal of Applied Microbiology.*

Wang, L.G., et al.(1991). *Determination of DNA Topoisomerase II Activity for Screening Antitumor Agents.* Chung Kuo Yau Li Hsueh Pao.

Weyers, et al. (1989). Skin Absorption of Oils. Pharmacokinetics. *Pharm Unserer Zeit.*

Wie, M.B., et al. (1997). Eugenol in Clove Essential Oil Protects Brain Cells from Excitotoxic and Oxidative Injury. *Neuroscience Letter.*

Zanker, K.S., et al. (1980). Evaluation of Surfactant Effects of Essential Oils for Colds. Respiration.

CHAPTER 3: YOUR BLOOD TYPE MAKES THE RULES

Addi, G.J. (1959). Blood Groups in Acute Rheumatism. *Scottish Medical Journal, 4.*

Aird, E., et al. (1954). Relationship Between ABO Blood Groups and Cancer of *The Stomach. British Medical Journal, I.*

American Asso Blood Banks. (1990). (10th ed.). *Technical Manual.*

Atkins, R., R.W. Herwood. (1972). *Dr. Atkins' Diet Revolution.* New York: Bantam.

Boyd, W.C. (1950). *Genetics and Races of Man: Introduction to Modern Physical Anthropology.* Boston: Little Brown.

Brues, A.M. (1929). Test of Blood Group Selection. *American Journal of Forensic Medicine.*

D'Adamo, P. (1990). Gut Ecosystems III: The ABO and other Polymorphic Systems.

Townsend Letter for Doctors.

D'Adamo, P. (1990). Possible Alteration of ABO Blood Groups in Hodgkin's Lymphoma.
Journal of Naturopathic Medicine, I.

D'Adamo, P. (1991). *Gut Ecosystems II: Lectins and Other Mitogens.*
Townsend Letter to Doctors.

Freed, D.L.F. (1987). *Dietary Lectins and Disease.*
Food Allergy and Intolerance.

Gates, R.R. (1948). *Human Ancestry.* Cambridge, M.A. Harvard University Press.

Havlik, R., et al. (1969). Blood Groups and Coronary Heart Disease.
Lancet, Aug. 2.

Helm, R., A. Froese. (1981). Binding of Receptors by Various Lectins.
Int Arch Allergy Appl. *Immunology, 65.*

Kushi, M., A. Jack. (1983). *The Cancer Prevention Diet.* New York: St. Martin's.

Langkilde, N.C., et al. (1989). Binding of Wheat and Peanut Lectins to Human Cell Carcinoma. *Cancer: 64,4.*

Marcus, D.M. (1969). The ABO and Lewis Blood Group System.
New England Journal of Medicine.

Nachbar, M.S., et al. (1980). Lectins in the U.S. Diet: Isolation and Characterization.
American of Biological Chemistry, 255.

Nomi, T., A. Besher. (1983). *You are Your Blood Type.* New York: Pocket Renton, P.H., et al. (1962). Red Cells of All Four ABO Groups in a Case of Leukemia.
British Medical Journal, Feb 2.

Roberts, T.E., et al. (1988). Blood Groups and Lung Cancer.

British Journal of Cancer: 58,2.

Sheppard, P.M. (1959). Blood Groups and Natural Selection.

British Medical Bulletin,15.

Uimer, A.J., et al. (1982). Stimulation of Colony Formation of Human Lymphocytes by Wheat Germ Lectins. *Immunology, 47.*

CHAPTER 4: 3,000 YEAR OLD SECRET, OIL PULLING

Beck, J.D., et al. (1996). Periodontal disease and Cardiovascular Disease.

Periodontal, 67.

Billings, F. (1913). Focal infections as a Causative Factor in Chronic Arthritis.

J Am Med Assoc, 61.

Breiner, M.A. (1999). *Whole Body Dentistry.* Quantum Health Press.

Carter, C.B., et al. (1992). Severe Odogenic Infection Associated with Intravascular *Coagulation. Gen Dent, 40.*

Currie, W.J., V. Ho. (1993). Unexpected Death Asso with Acute Dentoalveolar Abscess. *Br J Oral Maxillofac Surg, 31.*

Cromie, W.J. (2002). Discovering Who Lives in Your Mouth, Clues to Cancer.

Harvard University Gazette, Aug. 22.

Cutler, A.H. (1999) *Amalgam Illness, Diagnosis and Treatment.*

Andrew Hall Cutler, Davidson, L.S.P., et al. (1949). Focal Infection in Rheumatoid Arthritis. *Ann Rheum Dis, 8.*

Fife, B. (2004). *The Coconut Oil Miracle.* (4th ed.). Avery Publishing.

Fife, B. (2008). *Oil Pulling Therapy.* Piccadilly Books ,Ltd.

Fife, B., (2013). *The Coconut Oil Miracle. (5th ed.).* Avery/Penguin Group (USA) LLC.

Groves, B. (2002). *Fluoride: Drinking Ourselves to Death.* New Leaf.

Huggins, H. (1993). *It's All in Your Head: Link Between Mercury Amalgams and Illness.* Avery Publishing.

Huggins, J. (2002). *Solving the MS Mystery: Help Hope, Recovery.* Matrix, Inc.

Hughes, R.A. (1994). Focal Infections Revisited. *Br J Rheumatol, 33.*

Hunter, W. (1900). Oral Sepsis as Cause of Disease. *Lancet, 215.*

Hunter, W. (1921). Coming of Age of Oral Sepsis. *British Medical Journal, 859.*

Kozarov, E.V., et al. (2005). Human Arteriosclerosis Plaque Contains Invasive Actinbacillus Gingivalis. *Arterioscler Thromb Vasc Biol, 25.*

Kraut, J.A., J.L. Hicks. (1976). Bacterial Endocarditis of Dental Origin. *J Oral Surg, 34.*

Kulacz, R., T.E. Levy. (2002). *The Roots of Disease: Connecting Dentistry to Medicine.* Xlibris, Corp.

Miller W.D. (1891). The Human Mouth as Focus of Infection. *Dental Cosmos, 33.*

Muhlestein, J.B. (2000). Chronic infection and Coronary Heart Disease. *Med Clin North Am, 84.*

Price, W.A. (1923). Dental Infections Vol 1 & 2. *Price-Pottenger Nutrition Foundation.*

Price, W.A. (2008). Nutrition and Physical Degeneration. (8th ed.). *Price-Pottenger Nutrition Foundation.*

Rosenow, E.C. (1921). Focal Infection and Localization of Bacteria. *Surg Gynecol Obstet, 33.*

Spaulding, C.R., J.M. Friedman. (1975). Bacterial Endocarditis secondary to Dental Infection.
New York Journal of Medicine, 41.

US Dept. Health and Human Services. (2000). *Oral Health in America: A Report of the Surgeon General. Rockville, MD.*

US Dept. of Health and Human Services. (2000) Nat'l Institute of Dental and Craniofacial *Research. National Institute of Health.*

Ziff, S. (1986). *Silver Dental Fillings: The Toxic Time Bomb.* Aurora Press.

CHAPTER 5: NATURE'S UNSUNG HERO, HYDROGEN PEROXIDE

Ackeman, N.B., F.B. rinkley. (1968). Comparison of Effects on Tissue Oxygenation of Hyperbaric Chamber and Intravascular Hydrogen Peroxide.
British Medical Journal (1985). Dec 14. pg 1706.

Cavanaugh, M. (2008). *The One-Minute Cure: Secret to Healing Virtually Any Disease.*
Think-Outside-the-Book Publishing, Inc.

Demarquay. (1886). *Essai Pneumatological Medicale. Paris. 637.*

Douglass, W.C. (1996). *Hydrogen Peroxide: Medical Miracle.*
Second Opinion Publishing, Inc.

Earth Clinic, LLc. (2008). *Hydrogen Peroxide Inhalation Method.*

Farr, C.H. (1987). *Journal of the American College for the Advancement of Medicine.*

Farr, C.H. (1987). The Therapeutic Use of Intravenous Hydrogen Peroxide.
Genesis Med Center, OK.

Finney J.W., et al. (1966). *Angiology, 17.*

Finney, J.W., B.E. Jay, G.J. Race, et al. (1966). Removal of Cholesterol from Human Atheromatous Arteis by Dilute Hydrogen Peroxide. *Angology, 17.*

Finney, J.W., G.A. Bella, G.J. Race, et al. (1965). Peripheral Blood Changes in Humans Following the Infusion of Hydrogen Peroxide into Carotid Artery. *Angio, 16.*

Grotz, W. Education Concerns for Hydrogen Peroxide (ECHO).
Newsletter on Oxygen Therapy, Delano, MN Hydrogen Peroxide Release from Human Platelets. (1982).

Biochimica et Biophysica Acta, 718.

Hydrogen Peroxide Mediated Killing of Bacteria. (1982).
Molecular and Cellular Biochemistry, 49.

Hydrogen Peroxide as a Remedial Agent. (1988).
Journal of the American Medical Asso, Vol X, No. 9, 262.
Interferon (IFN). (1983). *Journal of Interferon Research Vol 3,143.*

Journal of American Medical Association. April 11,1914. Killing of Blood-Stage Murine Malaria Parasites by Hydrogen Peroxide.
(1983). *Infection and Immunity, 456.*

Lebedev, L.V., A.O. Levin, M.P. Romankova, et al. (1984). Regional Oxygenation in Treatment of Severe Forms of Obliterating Diseases of Extremity Arteries.
Vstn Khir,132.

McCabe, E. (2003). *Flood Your Body with Oxygen.* (6th ed.). Energy Publications.

Nathan, C.F., Z.A. Cohn. (1981). *Journal of Experimental Medicine, 154.*

Nathan, C.F., Z.A. Cohen. (1985). Antitumor Effect of Hydrogen Peroxide.
Exp. Med., 154.

Oliver, T.H., B.C. Cantab. (1920). Influenzal Pneumonia: Intravenous Injection of
Hydrogen Peroxide. *Lancet, 142.*

Oya, Y., K. Yamamoto, A. Tonomura. (1986). Biological Activity of Hydrogen Peroxide.
Mutat Res, 172(3).

Root, R.K. J. Metcalf, N. Oshino, et al. (1975). H2O2 Release from Human Granulocytes
During Phagocytosis. *J Clinical Invest, 55.*

Rowley and Halliwell. (1983). *Clinical Science, 64.*

Shenep, J.L., D.C. Stokes, W.T. Hughes. (1985). Lack of Bacterial Activity after IV Hydrogen Peroxide in Experimental E. Coli Sepsis. *Infect Immun, 48.*

Singh, et al. (1940). *The Lancet,* May 18.

Urschel, H.C., J.W. FinneyA.R. Morale, et al. (1965). Cardiac Resuscitation with Hydrogen Peroxide. *Circ. (suppl II):* 31.

Urschel Jr., H.E. (1967). Cardiovascular Effects of Hydrogen Peroxide. *Dis. of Chest, 51.*

Warburg, O. Two-time Nobel Laureate. *The Prime Cause and Prevention of Cancer.*
Lecture: Lake Constance, Germany, June 30, 1966.

Williams, D. (2003). *The Many Benefits of Hydrogen Peroxide.* Lecture.

CHAPTER 6: ARE YOUR TEETH KILLING YOU?

Beck, J.D., et al. (1996). Periodontal disease and Cardiovascular Disease.

Periodontal, 67.

Billings, F. (1913). Focal infections as a Causative Factor in Chronic Arthritis.
J Am Med Assoc, 61.

Breiner, M.A. (1999). *Whole Body Dentistry.* Quantum Health Press.

Carter, C.B., et al. (1992). Severe Odogenic Infection Associated with Intravascular Coagulation. *Gen Dent, 40.*

Currie, W.J., V. Ho. (1993). Unexpected Death Asso with Acute Dentoalveolar Abscess. *Br J Oral Maxillofac Surg, 31.*

Cromie, W.J. (2002). Discovering Who Lives in Your Mouth, Clues to Cancer.
Harvard University Gazette, Aug. 22.

Cutler, A.H. (1999) *Amalgam Illness, Diagnosis and Treatment.* Andrew Hall Cutler.

Davidson, L.S.P., et al. (1949). Focal Infection in Rheumatoid Arthritis.
Ann Rheum Dis, 8.

Fife, B. (2008). *Oil Pulling Therapy.* Piccadilly Books ,Ltd.

Fischer, M.H. (1940). *Death and Dentistry.* Charles C. Thomas.

Huggins, H. (1993). *It's All in Your Head: Link Between Mercury Amalgams and Illness.* Avery Publishing.

Huggins, H.A., (2002). *Solving the MS Mystery: Help Hope, Recovery.* Matrix, Inc.

Hughes, R.A. (1994). Focal Infections Revisited. *Br J Rheumatol, 33.*

Hunter, W. (1900). Oral Sepsis as Cause of Disease. *Lancet, 215.*

Hunter, W. (1921). Coming of Age of Oral Sepsis. *British Medical Journal, 859.*

Kozarov, E.V., et al. (2005). Human Arteriosclerosis Plaque contains Invasive Actinbacillus Gingivalis. *Arterioscler Thromb Vasc Biol, 25.*

Kraut, J.A., J.L. Hicks. (1976). Bacterial Endocarditis of Dental Origin. *J Oral Surg, 34.*

Kulacz, R., T.E. Levy. (2002). *The Roots of Disease: Connecting Dentistry to Medicine.*
Xlibris, Corp.

Lewin, L. (1962) *Gifte und Vergiftungen (Health Consequences of Amalgam Fillings.)*

Meinig, G.E. (2008). *The Root Canal Cover Up.* Price Pottenger Nutrition.

Miller W.D. (1891). The Human Mouth as Focus of Infection. *Dental Cosmos, 33.*

Muhlestein, J.B. (2000). Chronic infection and Coronary Heart Disease.
Med Clin North Am, 84.

Price, W.A. (1923). *Dental Infections Vol 1 & 2.* Price-Pottenger Nutrition Foundation.

Price, W.A. (2008). *Nutrition and Physical Degeneration.* (8th ed.).
Price-Pottenger Nutrition Foundation.

Rosenow, E.C. (1921). Focal Infection and Localization of Bacteria. *Surg Gynecol Obstet, 33.*

Spaulding, C.R., J.M. Friedman. (1975). Bacterial Endocarditis Secondary to Dental Infection.
New York Journal of Medicine, 41.

Stock, A. (1950). Biography: Research on Amalgam Fillings. *Chem Berichte.*

Stock, A., E. Jaensch. (1983). Nothing New Under the Sun: Experiences with Mercury Poisoning. *Journal of Orthomolecular Psychiatry, 12(3).*

US Dept. Health and Human Services. (2000). *Oral Health in America: A Report of the Surgeon General.* Rockville, MD.

US Dept. of Health and Human Services. *(2000) Nat'l Institute of Dental and Craniofacial*

Research. National Institute of Health.

Ziff, S. (1986). *Silver Dental Fillings: The Toxic Time Bomb.* Aurora Press.

CHAPTER 7: REVERSING ALZHEIMER'S, THE SECRET KEY

Bishop, N.A., T. Lu., B.A. Yankner. (2010). Neural Mechanisms of Cognitive Decline.
Insight.

Bou, K.J., J.M. Rho. (2007). Anticonvulsant Mechanisms of Ketogenic Diet.
Epilepsia Vol 48, No 1.

Bu, G. (2009). Apolipoprotein E. and its Receptors in Alzheimer's Disease.
Natural Review Neuroscience Vol 10, No 5.

Cahill, G.F. Jr. (2006). Fuel Metabolism in Starvation. *Annu Rev Nutr Vol 26.*

Gilbert, G.L., P.L. Pyzik, J.M. Freedman. (2000). The Ketogenic Diet, Seizure Control.
Journal Child Neurology Vol 15.

Cahill, G.F. Jr., T.T. Aoki. (1980). *Alternate Fuel Utilization by Brain. Cerebral Metabolism and Neural Function.* William and Wilkins.

Caregiver Reports. coconutketones.com CunaneS., S. NugentM. Roy, et al. (2011). Brain Fuel Metabolism, Aging and Alzheimers.
Nutrition Vol 27, No1.

Fife, B., (2013). *The Coconut Oil Miracle.* *(5th ed.).* Avery/Penguin Group (USA) LLC.

Folstein, M.F., S.E. Folstein, P.R. McHugh. (1975). Mini Mental State: A Practical Method for Grading the Cognitive State of Patients for the Clinician. *J Psychiat Res Vol 12.*

Hartman, A.L., M. Gasior, E.P.G. Vinning, et al. (2007). Neuropharmacology of the Ketogenic Diet. *Pediatr Neurol Vol 36, No 5.*

Henderson, S.T. (Inventor). *Medium Chain Triglycerides for Treatment and Prevention of Alzheimer's Disease and Other Diseases Resulting from Reduced Neuronal Metabolism.*

U.S. Patent # 20080009467.

Henderson, S.T., (2008). Ketone Bodie as Therapeutic Treatment of Alzheimer's Disease.

Journal of the American Society for Experimental NeuroTherapeutics Vol 5.

Hashim, S.A., S. Bergen, Jr., K. Krell, et al. (1964). Intestinal Absorption and Mode of Transport in the Portal Vein of Medium Chain Fatty Acids. *J Clin Invest Vol 43.*

Hoyer, S. (1991). Abnormalities of Glucose Metabolism in Alzheimer's Disease.
Ann NY Acad Sci Vol 640.

Hoyer, S. (2000). Brain Glucose Metabolism Abnormalities in Alzheimer's Disease, Causes and Consequences. *Exp Gerontol Vol 35.*

Huttenlocher, P.R.A.J. Wilbourn, J.M. Signore. (1971). Medium Chain Triglycerides as Therapy for Childhood Epilepsy. *Neurology Vol 21.*

Itzhaki, R.F., M.A. Wozniak. (2008). Herpes Simplex Virus 1 In Alzheimer's Disease:
The Enemy Within. *J Alzheimer's Dis Vol13.*

Knopp, R.H., B.M. Retzlaff. (2004). Saturated Fat Prevents Coronary Heart Disease.

American Journal of Clinical Nutrition Vol 80.

Mauer, K., S. Volk, H. Gerbaldo. (1997). August D and Alzheimer's Disease.

Lancet.Vol 349.

Newport, M.T. (2011). *Alzheimer's Disease What if There Was a Cure?*

Basic Health Publications, Inc.

Owen, O.E. (2005). Ketones Bodies as a Fuel for the Brain During Starvation.

Biochem Mol Biol Educ Vol 33, No 4.

Page, K.A., A. Williamson, N. Yu, et al. (2009). Medium Chain Fatty Acids Improve Cognitive Function in Typei Diabetic Patients. Diabetes Vol 58, No 5.

Prins, M.L. (2008). Ketogenic Diet as Treatment of Neurotrauma. Epilepsia Vol 49.

Prins, M.L. (2008). Cerebral Ketone Metabolism after Brain Injury.

J Cereb Blood Flow Metab Vol 18.

Pior, I.A., F. Davidson, C.E. Salmond et al. (1981). T*he Pukapuka and Tokelau Island Studies:*

Cholesterol, Coconuts, Diets on Poynesian Atolls.

Progress Report on Alzheimer's Disease. (2009). *National Institute of Health/National Institute on Aging/Alzheimer's Disease Education and Referral Center.*

Small, G.W., L.M. Ercoli, D.H.S. Silverman, et al. (2000). Cerebral and Metabolic Decline in Persons at Risk for Alzheimer's Disease. *PNAS Vol 97, No 11.*

St. Ong, M.P., A. Bosarge, L.L.T. Goree, et al. (2008). Medium Chain Triglyceride Oil Consumption as Part of Weight Loss Diet Does Not lead to Adverse Metabolic Effects.

Journal of the American College of Nutrition Vol 27, No 5.

Taha, A.Y., S.T. Henderson, W.M. Burnham. (2009). Dietary Enrichment with Medium ChainTriglycerides/Treating Age-Related Cognitive Decline. *Neurochem Res Vol 34, No 9.*

Tantibhehyangkul, P., S.A. Hashim. (1975). Medium Chain Triglycerides Feeding in Premature Infants. *Pediatrics Vol 55.*

U.S. Dept. of Agriculture Nutrient Data Laboratory. (2010). *Nutrient Analysis of Coconut Oil.* usda.gov/nutrientdata.

Veech, R.L. (2004). Therapeutic Implications and Effects of Ketone Bodies in Pathological Conditions. *Prostaglandins, Leukot Essential Fatty Acids Vol 70.*

CHAPTER 8: BUDWIG PROTOCOL CANCER TREATMENT

Budwig, J. (1957). International Congress of Nutrition Symposium. Paris, France.

Budwig, J. (2008). *Cancer: The Problem and the Solution.* NexusGmbh.

Budwig, J. (2010). *The Budwig Cancer & Coronary Heart Disease Prevention Diet.* Freedom Press.

Budwig, J. (2018). *Flax Oil as a True Aid Against Arthritis, Heart Infarction, Cancer and Other Diseases. (3rd ed.).* Apple Publishing.

Budwig, J. (2018).(3rd. ed.). *The Oil Protein Diet Cookbook.* Apple Publishing.

Edwards, G. I. (1990). *Biology the Easy Way, 2ndEdition, Barron's Educational Series Inc.*

Edwards, G.I. (2021) *Complete Guide to Biology.* Barron's Educational Services.

Escher, U., G. Wei. (2011). *A Day in the Budwig Diet: Home Healing Protocol Against Cancer.* Create Space Independent Publishing Platform.

Ley, B.M. (1998). *The Forgotten Nutrient MSM: On our Way Back to Health with Sulfur* BL Publications.

Paustian, T. (2003). *Cell Wall.*

Verma, O.P. (2014). *Cancer Cause and Cure: A Book on Budwig Protocol.*
Create Space Independent Publishing Platform.

Verma, O.P. (2019). *Budwig Protocol: Documented 90% Success.*
Independently published.

Warburg, O. Two-time Nobel Laureate. *The Prime Cause and Prevention of Cancer.*
Lecture: Lake Constance, Germany, June 30, 1966.

CHAPTER 9: CLEAN OUT YOUR ARTERIES, CARDIO PROTEGEN

Cooke, J.P., A.H. Singer, P. Tsao, et al. (1992). Antiatherogenic Effects of L-Arginine In Hypercholesterolemic Rabbits. *Journal of Clinical Investigation, 90.*

Fried, R., C. Woodson, J. Thornton. (1999). *The Arginine Solution.* Warner Books, Inc.

Hishikawa, K., T. Nakaki, h. Suzuki, et al. (1992). L-Arginine as an Antihypertensive Agent. *Journal of Cardiovascular Pharmacology, Supp 12, 20.*

Joint National Committee. (1998). Report on Detection, Evaluation and Treatment of

High Blood Pressure. *Archives of Internal Medicine, 148.*

Korbet, R., K. Bieron, R.J. Gryglewski. (1993). Effects of L-Arginine in Hypertensive
Patients with Hypercholesterolemia. *The New England Journal of Medicine, 328.*

Koshland, D.E. (1992). The Molecule of the Year. *Science, 258.*

Moncada, S., R.M.J. Palmer, E.A., Higgs. (1988). The Discovery of Nitric Oxide as
An Indogenous Nitrovasodilator. *Hypertension, 12.*

Moncada, S., E.A., Higgs. (1990). *Nitric Oxide from L-Arginine: A Bio-regulatory System.*
Amsterdam: Elsevier Science Publishers.

Nakaki, T., K. Hishikawa K., H. Suzuki, et al. (1990). L-Arginine Induced Hypotension.
The Lancet, 336.

Onish, D.M. (1990). *Dr. Dean Ornish's Program for Reversing Heart Disease.*
New York: Random House.

Rector, T.S., A.J. Bank, K.A. Mullen, et al. (1996). Randomized, Doble-Blind, Placebo-Controlled Study of Supplemental Oral L-Arginine in Patients with Heart Failure. *Circulation, 93.*

CHAPTER 10: CHARGING THE BATTERY OF LIFE, CELLFOOD

Budwig, J. (1957). International Congress of Nutrition Symposium. Paris, France.

Budwig, J. (2008). *Cancer: The Problem and the Solution.* NexusGmbh.

Levine, S.A. (1985). Antioxidant Adaptation. Free Radical Biochemistry.

Holden, D., PhD. (2021) Cell and Molecular Biology. Perelman School of Medicine.
University of Pennsylvania.

Warburg, O. Two-time Nobel Laureate. *The Prime Cause and Prevention of Cancer.*
Lecture: Lake Constance, Germany, June 30, 1966.

Made in the USA
Monee, IL
16 April 2023

31962514R10218